D0931969

COMMUNICATING IN THE CLINIC

Negotiating Frontstage and Backstage Teamwork

Health Communication
Gary L. Kreps, series editor

COMMUNICATING IN THE CLINIC

Negotiating Frontstage
and Backstage Teamwork

Laura L. Ellingson, Ph.D.
Santa Clara University

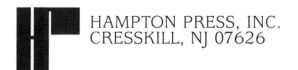

HAMPTON PRESS, INC.
CRESSKILL, NJ 07626

Copyright © 2005 by Hampton Press, Inc.

All rights reserved. No part of this publication may be reproduced, stored in a retrieval system, or transmitted in any form or by any means, electronic, mechanical, photocopying, microfilming, recording, or otherwise, without permission of the publisher.

Printed in the United States of America

Ellingson, Laura L.
    Communicating in the clinic : negotiating frontstage and backstage teamwork / Larua L. Ellingson.
        p. cm. -- (Health communication)
    Includes bibliographical references and indexes.
    ISBN 1-57273-599-6 -- ISBN 1-57273-600-3
        1. Health care teams. 2. Communication in medicine. I. Title. II. Health communication (Cresskill, N.J.)
    R729.5.H4E43 2004
    610.69--dc22

                                                        2004051480

Permission to include previously published material is gratefully acknowledged.

Ellingson, L. L. (2003). Interdisciplinary health care teamwork in the clinic backstage. *Journal of Applied Communication Research, 31*(2), 93-117. Copyright ©2003 National Communication Association.

Ellingson, L. L. (1998). Then you know how I feel: Empathy, identification, and reflexivity. *Qualitative Inquiry,* 492-514. Copyright ©1998 Sage Publication. Reprinted by permission of Sage Publication.

Hampton Press, Inc.
23 Broadway
Cresskill, NJ 07626

This book is dedicated to the remarkable team members, patients, and patients' companions of the Interdisciplinary Oncology Program for Older Adults. Although I have protected individuals' privacy with pseudonyms, I could never disguise my overwhelming admiration for all that you are and all that you accomplish together, nor my gratitude for all that you shared with me.

Contents

Acknowledgments

This book reflects the insights, inspiration, and support of a great number of colleagues, family, and friends. I am deeply grateful to many who have helped me along the way, some of whom are listed here.

Mary Tarrier Kleppinger was instrumental to my survival of cancer more than 15 years ago and has been a true friend, along with her family, ever since; I am forever blessed by her presence in my life. Patrice M. Buzzanell has been my feminist mentor and "advisor-for-life" since I began my master's program in 1995; my gratitude for her continues to grow as time passes. Patrice also introduced me to the wonderful members of the Organization for the Study of Communication, Language, and Gender, who continue to nurture me and who bestowed on me the honor of the 2002 Cheris Kramerae Dissertation Award for my dissertation, on which this book is based.

My doctoral committee members at the University of South Florida (USF) provided tremendous professional and research support; thanks to Arthur P. Bochner, Carolyn DiPalma, Eric M. Eisenberg, and Marsha L. Vanderford. Carolyn Ellis has been my mentor, dissertation advisor, and friend since a sad day in October 1997 that was redeemed by her warmth and brilliance; I will always be thankful for her guidance and encouragement. Many present and former members of the Department of Communication and the Women's Studies Department at USF have been faithful friends and wonderful colleagues. In particular, I am grateful to Bethany C. Goodier and Elizabeth Curry who read earlier drafts of this manuscript and gave me valuable feedback and encouragement; to Leigh Berger Serrie for our heartening chai chats during the initial draft writing; to Elena and Georgia Strauman who helped me work out innumerable practical and theoretical aspects of this project during our evening walks; to Sasha Normand who helped me to articulate my own feminist vision; and to Debbie Walker who always makes me laugh.

My current department members at Santa Clara University (SCU) are wonderful colleagues; special thanks to Sunwolf, Lisa Osteraas, and Connie Rice for helping me find my way. I am grateful to the members of the Women's Faculty Group and the Program for the Study of Women and Gender at SCU for providing me with a strong feminist community, and to the members of my research writing group for their encouragement and helpful editorial feedback.

I would like to express my deep appreciation to my series editor, Gary L. Kreps, who has been wonderfully patient, challenging me to do my very best and helping me in every way I needed. A million thanks to Barbara Bernstein at Hampton Press for her faith in my project and to Mariann Hutlak for her excellent work in shepherding my manuscript through the production process. For her assistance with the index for this book, I am grateful to my colleague Judith Perry.

A heartfelt thanks to all of my extended family and friends, but particularly my parents Jane and Larry LaPierre, my beloved auntie Joan BeJune, my brother and sister-in-law Jim and Brigitte LaPierre, and my nephew and niece Zachory and Jamie LaPierre—thank you for believing in me. For their boundless enthusiasm and encouragement, warm hugs to Kelly and the Friday night gang, my 6:15 am water aerobics buddies, and Matt and Mary Bell.

To the current and past IOPOA team members, patients, and companions who are the focus of this project: You amaze me, and I am grateful for the privilege of having known you.

Finally, I lovingly thank my best friend and partner Glenn Ellingson whose strength, love, and unshakable faith in me got me through the difficult parts of this project and helped me to celebrate the joyous ones.

1

SETTING THE (BACK)STAGE

An Introduction

I perch on the narrow window sill on the edge of the staff work area in the Southeast Regional Cancer Center[1] outpatient clinic and watch the health care providers as they go about their tasks. The fluorescent lights of the clinic make everyone look washed out, even olive-complexioned Dr. Gino Armani and latte-skinned nursing assistant Sheri Clarke. I shudder to think just how grayish my transplanted New England complexion looks in the harsh light. I have been observing the Interdisciplinary Oncology Program for Older Adults (IOPOA), an interdisciplinary program for cancer patients over the age of 70, for about half an hour this morning, and so far everything has been pretty routine.

Sheri ushers a patient onto the scale in the hallway and then into an examination room. Ashley Breton, registered dietitian, searches a patient chart for height and weight information that she adds to her dietary assessment form, and Elaine Lyndon jumps up from her chair, heading to the cart

---

[1] The names of the cancer center, oncology program, team members, patients, patients' companions, and all other incidental characters are pseudonyms used to protect the privacy of my research participants. I have also used pseudonyms for my personal physicians.

that holds new patients' charts. As nurse practitioner for the team, Elaine takes the medical history and does the physical exam before the patients see one of the oncologists. Sitting on a stool, Dr. Armani punches a series of buttons on a phone and spews forth information on an oncology patient into the hospital's computerized dictation system, his strong Italian accent making his rapid-fire speech difficult to understand. Still dictating, he waves when he notices me, and I give him a friendly wave back.

Glancing around to my left, I see Joyce Fitzgerald typing a social work assessment note on a patient at one of the computers. Another phone rings, and one of the clinic's administrative assistants moves quickly to answer it. I flatten myself against the wall and try to stay out of everyone's way. It is only 9:15 a.m., but the clinic is already in full swing. Technicians and nurses move up and down the hall, the photocopier beeps, and the laser printer whirs. Like a carefully coordinated, frenetic dance, the clinic hums with the constant motion of a myriad of health care providers and researchers working behind the scenes in the crowded, over-air-conditioned desk area. A short hallway of examination rooms extends out from the far side of the desk, ending with a door to the waiting room. Staff members enter the hallway to meet with patients and their loved ones, returning to document and discuss their findings.

The mix of sounds and quick movements makes it difficult for me to concentrate on any one person or conversation even after spending several hours a week for 2 years with the program. At least I am past the constant nausea that marked my early days in the clinic. As a cancer survivor, I find the ghosts of treatments past lurking everywhere—pamphlets on Adriamycin, a chemotherapy drug I took; charts, reports, and CAT scan images; hordes of white-coated people; the crinkle of stiff white paper on the examination table as a patient gingerly sits.

I see Elaine as she reaches the door to Room 3, where Mr. Lyons and his wife are waiting.

"Elaine, mind if I tag along?" I call out to her.

"Not at all. Come on," she says. I wait behind her as she knocks and opens the door. "Mr. Lyons?" she asks the large man who sits waiting. At his nod, she continues. "I'm Elaine Lyndon, the nurse practitioner with the team." She shakes hands with her patient and then turns to the woman sitting beside him. Offering her hand she asks, "And you are . . . ?"

"This is my wife, Elaine," chimes Mr. Lyons.

"Nice to meet you, Mrs. Lyons. And this is Laura," she adds, gesturing to me.

"Hi! It is so nice to meet you," I say, shaking hands with both of them. Mr. Lyons' hand is cold and clammy, and his skin has an unhealthy pallor. "I'm studying communication, and I would like to listen to how the staff communicates with you today, if that is all right with you?" I smile and shift my gaze between the patient and his wife.

"Well, that's just fine," says Mr. Lyons, nodding. I look at Mrs. Lyons, and she nods and smiles. Her blue eyes look anxious.

"Thank you very much. I will just stand over here out of the way," I say, moving to lean against the counter on the opposite side of the narrow room.

Elaine pulls a chair up to the end of the counter and spreads out her many forms, reports, and notes. "I am going to ask you a lot of questions, and then we'll do a brief exam, OK?"

"OK," replies Mr. Lyons. His shoulders droop, and he seems short of breath. Elaine zips through the list of past ailments, with Mr. Lyons responding yes or no and at times offering a date or other bit of information. When Elaine gets to the lifestyle questions, she asks casually, "No heavy alcoholism?"

Mr. Lyons shifts uncomfortably in his seat. "Well, I drink a lot of beer, but not as much as I used to." His eyes are moist, and he looks sad.

Elaine smiles gently at him and puts down her pen. "Mr. Lyons, we need to do a couple of tests. I am concerned about your heart. Have you been taking your heart medications?"

"No," he says quietly. "I just got so frustrated. None of my doctors would talk to each other, and they all put me on all these pills and then when I was in the hospital, they put me on some more. So finally, I just quit taking all of them. I figured I would wait until I saw the doctor today and hopefully he could straighten it all out."

"OK, well we need to give you an EKG and also monitor your pulse, OK?" says Elaine. It is not really a question, but more a statement of fact.

"OK, yeah," answers Mr. Lyons agreeably.

"Someone will be right in to see you," she says, heading out the door, her face grim. Outside the room, Elaine springs into action. "Beth," she calls as she walks down the hall toward the team's registered nurse. "Order a stat EKG for Mr. Lyons and also get a pulse monitor on him immediately, please." Nodding, Beth picks up the phone. Elaine joins Dr. Armani as he reviews a chart.

Concern evident on her face, team pharmacist Susan Day approaches me and asks, "What are they going to do about Mr. Lyons?"

"I don't know," I say. "But Elaine ordered a stat EKG."

"Good," she says. "He's a polypharmacy *nightmare*." Shaking her head, Susan adds, "We have to do something about his cardiac meds." She walks over to join Elaine and Dr. Armani's discussion.

"His blood pressure's sky high, his pulse is all over the place. He has urinary frequency, pain, and fatigue. He looks awful," Elaine says, searching Dr. Armani's face carefully. "I almost think we need to admit him." Dr. Armani nods.

Waving a sheet of paper, Susan demands, "Look at this list of drugs. It's a nightmare. He was taking double of some meds and then stopped taking them all suddenly because he didn't know what they were all for and he was frustrated."

Leaning over the counter, Ashley adds her thoughts on Mr. Lyons' nutritional profile. "He's not eating well. His weight is OK, but that is probably because he is drinking so much beer. He's not doing well at all." Ashley's voice is sad and yet somehow matter of fact at the same time.

"He could code at any minute, " points out Elaine, shaking her head as she reads the alarming results of Mr. Lyons's EKG and his wildly fluctuating pulse that Beth handed to her.

Joyce looks up from her computer screen. "He's very depressed; he definitely needs help. His score on the GDS [geriatric depression scale] was really high."

"OK," says Dr. Armani. "We should admit him." He is glancing through a stack of CAT scan images of Mr. Lyons's abdomen as the other team members talk to him.

Elaine asks Beth to call over to the main hospital for a bed. Abruptly, Elaine and Dr. Armani turn and proceed to Mr. Lyons's room; I'm hot on their heels.

"I'm Dr. Armani," says the doctor as he shakes hands with the Lyons. They both smile, and Dr. Armani gets right to the point. "Listen, Mr. Lyons. We need to admit you immediately. I think you have a blood disorder, and we will confirm that with a marrow test. But right now we must deal with your heart. Before we can do anything else, your heart *must* be under control. Your pulse is fluctuating between 55 and 120. It's very dangerous, OK?"

"Yes, I want it straightened out," says Mr. Lyons, his wife nodding silently.

"OK, we are making arrangements now," says Dr. Armani, standing. He places his large hand on Mr. Lyons's shoulder. "Someone will be back in a moment, OK?"

"OK," answers Mr. Lyons simply.

Dr. Armani nods and then exits the room quickly, Elaine and I following. Elaine says, "I think we should call an ambulance to take him over."

"No, they can drive over," responds Dr. Armani with a trace of impatience in his voice.

"No," says Beth vehemently. "We are liable. We need to get him an ambulance. Something could happen just in getting him across the street. We *have* to get an ambulance."

Elaine nods. Dr. Armani shrugs, then nods as well. Beth calls for an ambulance, then lets Mr. Lyons know that the EMTs are on their way. He looks anxious, but agrees to the plan.

I am worried about Mr. Lyons. His pain and frustration call to mind the many frustrations of my own illness, and I shiver with the memories. I hurriedly type notes on what is happening, caught up in the drama. The tiny keys of my palm top computer click as I try to get down the details. My fingers are still moving swiftly across the miniature keyboard 5 minutes later when the EMTs take Mr. Lyons away on a stretcher, his wife trailing behind.

I am trying to get it all down—how the team shares facts and opinions about patients, how the other team members contribute not only their expert knowledge, but persuasive tactics to influence the physician's decision, how concerned and yet calm everyone is.

"OK," says Elaine to Dr. Armani, shaking her head as if to rid it of troubling thoughts. "Are you ready for me to report on the next patient?"

Dr. Armani answers with slight impatience, "Yeah, yeah. Go ahead," and she begins her recitation of symptoms, signs, and surgeries.

I stop typing and stare at them in shock. I can't believe they are just moving on to the next patient. Yet despite the intensity of the crisis, there is no time to dwell on Mr. Lyons; the examination rooms are full of other patients waiting to be seen. The team members must be able to shift gears smoothly and resume the routine once they have done what they can for Mr. Lyons. I stand immobile, knowing they are doing what needs to be done. I am utterly unable to fathom how they manage to do it day in and day out.

STUDYING A TEAM IN ACTION

Incidents like the prior one are part of the daily world of the Interdisciplinary Oncology Program for Older Adults (IOPOA) at the Southeast Regional Cancer Center (SRCC). The IOPOA team consisted of two oncologists (one of whom is also the director of the program), a nurse practitioner, two registered nurses, a registered dietitian, a licensed clinical social worker, a clinical pharmacist, and an administrative assistant (she worked in an office suite apart from the clinic and served a number of support functions). The team provided comprehensive geriatric assessment and treatment recommendations to each new patient over the age of 70 who came to SRCC for treatment or a second opinion. Patients underwent a thorough medical history, a physical exam, and a psychosocial evaluation. Additionally, each new patient was screened for depression, cognitive processing deficits, risk of polypharmacy (overmedication or drug interactions), physical impairment or disability, and malnutrition. All of these assessments affected the treatment plans that the oncologists developed. As team members cycled through each of the patient's rooms (typically three patients were scheduled simultaneously), they communicated with each other (and other cancer center personnel) in the halls and desk area.

A health care team is "a group of people, often from different disciplines, who work collaboratively with the specific purpose of delivering better care to clients" (Kreps & Thornton, 1992, p. 82). Multidisciplinary and interdisciplinary health care teams continue to grow in popularity in virtually all aspects of health care, but particularly in the field of geriatrics, where comprehensive assessment by a team is well established as a necessary and beneficial aspect of health care delivery (Rubenstein, Stuck, Siu, & Wieland, 1991). Geriatric teams are designed to meet the needs of elderly patients through comprehensive geriatric assessment. Older patients are likely to have co-morbidities (multiple illnesses) and fragmented care, seeing a different specialist for each chronic or acute condition and greatly increasing the need for coordination of care and treatment (Beisecker, 1996). Additionally, significant attention to patients' "lifeworld" (i.e., to aspects of their lives beyond their medical diagnoses and treatment; Mishler, 1984) is critical to the care of older patients because of the unique biopsychosocial, financial, and relational factors that often confront people in their later years (Estes, 1981; Mellor, Hyer, & Howe, 2002).

The vast majority of studies of health care teams have sought to establish correlations between team approaches to care and measurable patient outcomes.[2] Interdisciplinary teams often improve overall care for patients (Cooke, 1997; Cooley, 1994; Fagin, 1992; McHugh, West, Assatly, Duprat et al., 1996; Pike, 1991; Wieland, Kramer, Waite, & Rubenstein, 1996), and promote job satisfaction for team members (Abramson & Mizrahi, 1996; Gage, 1998; McHugh et al., 1996; Pike, 1991; Resnick, 1997; Siegel, 1994).[3] Multidisciplinary teams can facilitate and improve training of students in medicine, nursing, and allied health fields, as well as enable veteran staff to learn from each other (Abramson & Mizrahi, 1996; Edwards & Smith, 1998; Turner, Sheldon, Coles, Mountford, Hillier, Radway, & Wee, 2000). Geriatric evaluation teams are particularly effective at assessment and intervention (Applegate, Miller, Graney et al., 1990; McCormick, Inui, & Roter, 1996; Rubenstein, Josephson, & Wieland et al., 1984).

---

[2]Specifically, multidisciplinary and interdisciplinary team care has been associated with the following outcomes: decrease in length of hospital stay (Barker, Williams, Zimmer, Van Buren et al., 1985; Wieland, Kramer, Waite, & Rubenstein, 1996); nurse perceptions of good quality patient care (Trella, 1993); increased patient satisfaction (Trella, 1993); better coordination of patient care (McHugh et al., 1996); increased use of hospital rehabilitation services (Schmitt, Farrell, & Heinemann, 1988); improved functioning in "Activities of Daily Living" (Rubenstein, Abrass, & Kane, 1981; Rubenstein, Josephson, Wieland, English et al., 1984; Rubenstein, Wieland, English, Josephson et al., 1984); improved pain control (Trella, 1993); decreased emergency room usage (Rubenstein, Josephson, Wieland, English et al., 1984); fewer nursing home admissions following hospitalization (Wieland et al., 1996; Zimmer, Groth-Junker, & McClusker, 1985); decreased mortality 1 year after discharge (Langhorne, Williams, Gilchrist, & Howie, 1993; Rubenstein et al., 1991; Wieland et al., 1996); decreased prescribing of psychotropic drugs among nursing home residents (Schmidt, Claesson, Westerholm, Nilsson, & Svarstad, 1998); and decreased overall health care costs (Williams, Williams, Zimmer, Hall, & Podgorski, 1987).

[3]Institutional context heavily influences team effectiveness (Opie, 1997; Siegel, 1994). Because hospitals are concerned with insurance reimbursement, administrators pressure teams to define services with a great deal of specificity. The essential caregiving function of many staff members is difficult to define and hence impossible to be paid for (Estes, 1981).

Despite the correlations between teams, desired patient outcomes, and employee satisfaction, we know relatively little about day-to-day health care team communication practices (Opie, 1997). Research on actual team communication is limited, and it has been primarily analyses of formal team meetings (for an excellent study of team meetings, see Opie, 2000). Much of the research on teams is "anecdotal, exhortatory and prescriptive . . . there is an absence of research describing and analyzing teams in action" (Opie, 1997, p. 260; see also Mizrahi & Abramson, 1994; Sands, 1993; Sheppard, 1992). Moreover, theorists of teamwork have noted significant problems with the organization, training (or lack of training), socialization, and management of health care teams that need to be addressed before teamwork can be optimally effective (Bateman, Bailey, & McLellan, 2003; Clark, 1994; McClelland & Sands, 1993; Opie, 1997; Saltz, 1992).[4] Clearly, there are significant problems with teamwork, and exploration of communication on real teams (rather than only measuring patient outcomes) is needed. Documentation and explication of existing communication practices on teams will help generate strategies for improving communication.

To complement existing research by focusing on explicating team processes rather than measuring outcomes, I undertook an ethnography (participant observation) of an interdisciplinary team in a clinical setting. Qualitative research that looks at communication and the meanings constructed in communication, rather than strictly outcomes, is crucial to improving medical practice and bringing more voices into the medical world (Miller & Crabtree, 2000). Rather than focusing on team meetings as the primary site of teamwork, I chose instead to concentrate on the plethora of fleeting interactions in "backstage" clinic areas that together constitute dynamic teamwork.

Based on my ethnographic fieldwork with the IOPOA team, I determined that the conceptualization of teamwork provided by existing theory and research was inadequate to explain some crucial aspects of teamwork. I developed three claims about teamwork in health care settings that form the foundation of this book:

---

[4]Opie (1997) summarizes the problems of team work as follows:

> inadequate, or an absence of, organisational support; the absence of training in team work; the absence of orientation programmes for new members joining the team; lack of interprofessional trust resulting in complicated power relations between professionals; an overabundance or, alternatively, an absence of conflict; lack of clear structures and directions; unclear goals; the dominance of particular discourses resulting in the exclusion of others; the existence of tensions between professional discourses resulting in potentially unsafe practices; lack of continuity of members; difficulty of definition of key terms; the production of client discussions which, far from addressing client goals, marginalise them and contribute to clients' disempowerment; and an absence of teams' examination of their processes. (p. 262)

◄ Teamwork must be recognized as taking place outside of designated team meetings, through informal communication channels, and in dyads and triads of team members, rather than as primarily occurring within full team meetings.

◄ Backstage team communication (communication among team members without patients present) is interwoven intricately with frontstage (health care provider-patient communication); the boundaries between these are fluid and permeable, not sharply delineated as they are currently theorized.

◄ Team communication is heavily constrained and shaped by persistent gender, racial, class, and disciplinary hierarchies in the medical establishment; structural and individual inequalities are not natural, neutral, or inevitable, and they are integral to the daily enactment of teamwork through communication.

Underlying these claims is a methodological critique of the relationship between how teamwork research generally is conducted and what kinds of knowledge are subsequently produced (or suppressed) in such research. The focus of most team research on formal meetings, the conceptual bifurcation of provider-patient communication from interdisciplinary communication, and the obscuring of the effects of power and hierarchy on team communication are not incidental; they reflect the history of modern health care delivery and research.

THEORETICAL PERSPECTIVE

I have used the term *backstage* to refer to the staff-only areas of the clinic where preparation for and documentation of visits with patients are done. Before going further, I want to introduce Goffman's theorizing of the backstage sphere and its meaning for interpersonal communication. In his classic work, *The Presentation of Self in Everyday Life*, Goffman (1959) presented a view of communication using a performance metaphor:

> A "performance" can be defined as all the activity of a given participant on a given occasion which serves to influence in any way any of the other participants. . . . The pre-established pattern of action which is unfolded during a performance and which may be presented or played through on other occasions may be called a "part" or a "routine." (Goffman, 1959, pp. 15-16)

According to Goffman, we are always playing one or more roles. Often the roles we play are part of a group, or team, performance. A particular definition of a setting or situation and the performance is often dependent on the agreement on the definition of the situation and subsequent performances by others; a bond of "reciprocal dependence" exists to keep the show going. Goffman defined a *team* as "any set of individuals who co-operate in staging a single routine" (p. 79). That cooperation is accomplished through communication; as team members communicate, they socially construct the meaning of teamwork. Indeed, "Communication is not just a tool that groups use; groups are best regarded as a phenomenon that emerges from communication" (Frey, 1994, p. x).

The team's performance involves a division between the frontstage and the backstage. The *front* is where a performance takes place. It consists of the setting, which is all of the furniture, equipment, and physical space that form the context for the performance, and the *personal front*, which includes all aspects of a person's appearance and manner—clothes, insignia, gender, race, age, gestures, and voice. Because the team members cooperated before their audience of patients and patient companions (in the frontstage), they necessarily had a view of each other as being "in the know" about how the performance is staged. Hence, the team did not continue the same performance when away from the audience (in this case, the patients and their companions). The area away from the audience is called the *backstage*:

> a place, relative to a given performance, where the impression fostered by the performance is knowingly contradicted as a matter of course. . . .
> It is here that the capacity of a performance to express something beyond itself may be painstakingly fabricated; . . . illusion and impressions are openly constructed. Here stage props and items of personal front can be stored in a kind of compact collapsing of whole repertoires of actions and characters. (Goffman, 1959, p. 112)

Goffman pointed out that the frontstage and backstage are usually adjacent so that performers can go back and forth, and performers expect that the audience will not enter the backstage. This was the case with the suite of examination rooms and the desk area, which were divided by a doorway. Due to concerns over patient confidentiality and security of records, patients were confined to their examination rooms and quickly redirected if they attempt to move into the backstage area. Because they have control over the setting (the delineation of areas in which patients can and cannot go), teams have control over the amount of information to which their audience (the patients) have access.

However, as Goffman pointed out, although some areas get labeled as front or backstage, "there are many regions which function at one time and in one sense as a front region and at another time and in another sense as a back region" (p. 126). Indeed, while the team dropped its performance of "health care professional/team member" designed for the patients (and patients' companions) and talked in the backstage emotionally and critically about patients, a performance of another type continued. Even when not performing for the patient audience, team members sought to maintain certain impressions of themselves to other team mates as, for example, reliable, competent, or friendly. As the team communicated in the backstage, they performed interdisciplinary collaboration to each other. Team members also performed their discipline, gender, and culture to each other, in addition to their particular personalities. Butler (1997) pointed out that people tend to think of their gender and ethnicity as inherent to their selves; however, gender and other social identities are constituted through repeated performance of and reinforcement for particular behaviors. Although team members seemed quite conscious of the performative nature of their communication with patients, they did not seem to conceptualize their backstage communication with each other as also performative. However, "The unthinking ease with which performers consistently carry off such standard maintaining routines does not deny that a performance has occurred, merely that the participants have been aware of it" (Goffman, 1959, p. 75).

My attention to the team's performance and its position within the medical system is in keeping with a "bona fide group" approach to studying small-group communication (Putnam & Stohl, 1990). Bona fide groups are natural occurring groups that have stable, but permeable, boundaries and are interdependent with their context (Putnam & Stohl, 1990). Putnam (1994) urged researchers of bona fide groups to pay close attention to "what is covert, implicit, and assumed normal" to reveal the deep structures of the group or team. Frey (1994), Poole (1990, 1994), and other communication scholars have championed a bona fide approach to enrich the conceptualization of small-group communication through exploration of groups in real-life contexts, rather than researcher-constructed, zero-history groups. By observing a real team in action, I was able to break out of the conceptual box that envisioned interdisciplinary collaboration as a process located primarily in formal team meetings and explore the dynamic structure of collaboration in the clinic developed among the IOPOA team members.

ETHNOGRAPHY

Ethnography is an ideal methodology to construct a detailed description of teamwork dynamics. Also called *participant observation* or *fieldwork*, ethnography involves careful observation that is documented in extensive fieldnotes (Lindlof & Taylor, 2002). Ethnographic methods offer several benefits over experimental, quantitative, or highly structured qualitative data-collection methods. First, ethnography allows researchers to look at both practitioners and patients together, instead of separating them for analysis. Beisecker (1990) explained that, "Too often, however, a researcher has focused either on patients or physicians, neglecting the relational aspects of the encounter. Any interaction between two persons is reflexive. The parties take cues from each other" (p. 19). Participant observation enables me to observe interactions among patients, patients' companions, a variety of health care providers, and myself.

Second, fieldwork is a qualitative method that allowed me to look holistically at content, process, language, and behavior in a medical context, rather than simply identifying or counting types of communicative practices of patients, physicians, or other health care providers from taped interactions or transcripts (Adelman, Greene, Charon, & Friedmann, 1990). Much research on teams and small groups has used researcher-produced groups because they allow for careful control of variables (Frey, 1994; Poole, 1994; Propp & Kreps, 1994). In turn this enables precise measurement of differences across groups. Such research generally supports a positivist (or postpositivist) approach to scientific inquiry in which control, measurement, detachment, reliability, and validity are highly valued (Frey, 1994). Such scientific goals were (and, in some cases, still are) presented as neutral and natural, rather than as reflecting and privileging specific approaches to defining and generating knowledge that emerged during the 18th-century Enlightenment movement (i.e., discovering objective knowledge of the world via the scientific method; Gergen, 1994; Haraway, 1988). In my research on a bona fide group, I privileged a different set of values more traditionally associated with femininity—connection with research participants, attention to the positionality (identity and roles) of the researcher, awareness of the indeterminacy of language, acknowledgment of the constructed nature of all knowledge, and interrogation of power dynamics (Meyers & Brashers, 1994; Reinharz, 1992). Such a qualitative and interpretive approach not only acknowledges the messiness of the research process, but considers it indispensable to understanding how communication happens in the real world. Conceptualizing the manner in which teams socially construct the processes and meanings of teamwork is not a task that lends itself to controlled studies (Putnam & Stohl, 1990).

My fieldnotes not only documented the conversational topics, they also recorded details of dress, mannerisms, tone, and emotion. I also observed interactions in a variety of settings. Almost all studies of health care teams have looked at weekly team rounds (meetings), where the team members meet to report information and make decisions; few have examined how team members interact outside of these meetings (Cott, 1998). My project involved observing team members with patients, within backstage clinic areas, in meetings, and in social settings. By interacting with IOPOA staff in multiple settings, I learned more about their communication styles and the effects of context on how they relate to each other and to me. For example, I went out for drinks after work with the team dietitian and social worker and a group of their friends, and I gained insight into the context of their lives outside the team.

Third, ethnography enabled me to study the workings of a health care team "in action" (Opie, 1997; Sands, 1993; Sheppard, 1992). Participant observation afforded me the opportunity to observe and converse with team members, patients, and caregivers as they went about providing and receiving health care. Sands (1993) advocated use of an ethnographic approach to teams "because of its capacity to uncover, through a prolonged engagement with a culture, the perspectives of the participants" (p. 548) as they engage in their work. Moreover, ethnographic studies of daily work on health care teams generate valuable insights as to what areas remain unexamined and in need of study (Allen, Griffiths, Lyne, Monoghan, & De Murphy, 2002).

My commitment to feminist theory and practice is part of an overall awareness of the construction of ethnography in a postmodern climate where positivism (strict belief in objectivity and the scientific method) has been radically challenged and innovative qualitative and critical approaches to ethnography and representation embraced (Denzin, 1997; Van Maanen, 1988). Although early ethnographers insisted on the objectivity of their observations and evaluations of the natives (Tedlock, 1991; Van Maanen, 1988), ethnographers now acknowledge (to varying degrees) their influence on their participants and the importance of exploring the nature of knowledge generated through participant observation (Behar, 1996; Tedlock, 1991). Rather than researcher neutrality, most contemporary ethnographers have the goal of careful attention to and reflection on the researcher's self in relation to participants (Denzin & Lincoln, 2000). I used my insights about my particular viewpoint and experiences as one aspect of my data (Ellingson, 1998).

As a feminist researcher, I was also highly cognizant of and interested in power dynamics. Although there are many definitions of feminism and feminist research methods (Reinharz, 1992), my approach to feminist research (as distinguished from other types of research methods) involves being acutely aware of power—who has it, how they got it, how it is used, what it does, how it is revealed and obscured in discourse, and how I, as a researcher, reify and/or resist it. For a more detailed discussion of feminist ethnographic practices, please see Appendix B.

My social privilege affects how I construct the meaning(s) of the IOPOA team, its medical context, and my role as a researcher. I want to point out some of the aspects of my position that specifically affect my understanding of the IOPOA team and its communication. I am a Euro-American, heterosexually partnered, middle-class woman who has earned a Ph.D. My gender, ethnicity, sexual orientation, education level, and age are very similar to that of the majority of the group I studied; I am culturally far more like the members of the IOPOA team than different. Of the 12 team members with whom I spent time in the clinic, 9 were White middle-class women raised in the United States. Half of the team members had attained a master's or higher level of education, and all had bachelor's degrees. The oncologists were from Western Europe. Although they certainly have cultural experiences and beliefs not held by the others, their communication styles did not differ significantly from the other team members. Ten of the 12 team members were married or in committed heterosexual partnerships.

Nevertheless, my identity as a cancer survivor set me apart from the team members. I survived osteogenic sarcoma (bone cancer) 15 years ago. I now live with an impaired and disfigured right leg following the removal of the tumor in my femur and subsequent reconstructive surgeries. Swelling, a 22-inch scar, a bulging muscle graft covered with a skin graft, an assortment of smaller scars, somewhat impaired mobility (e.g., difficulty negotiating staircases), and a limp mark me as *patient* to both the patients and staff. During the process of researching and writing this project, I went through removal of my gallbladder, orthoscopic surgery on my knee, two total knee replacements, and two surgeries to replace a broken bone graft with a titanium implant. My continual treatment ensured that I remember what it feels like to be a patient. I even got a sense of what it is like to be a patient at the SRCC because my surgeon at the time of my fieldwork moved his practice there several months before my first knee replacement surgery.

Because my sense of identification with both the team and the patients was strong, and I participated in the clinic as a researcher (i.e., as neither a geriatric patient nor an actual team member), I had a dynamic view of the clinic. I empathized with the constraints of each role and endeavored to experience both a personal connection to and a detached view of the team members, patients, and patients' companions. The opportunities and constraints of my cancer-survivor-as-ethnographer identity is explored in the autoethnographic account in chapter 4 (see also Ellingson, 1998).

Some scholars and professionals, particularly those schooled in positivist research methods that stress objectivity, control, measurement, and generalizability, may find it difficult or uncomfortable to make sense of ethnographic research findings that seem subjective. Interpretive research methods are designed to produce "thick description" (Geertz, 1973) of naturally occurring phenomena through the construction of richly detailed accounts that shed light on the complexities of daily communication. Findings such as those presented here are meant to complement positivist research by providing a more holistic perspective, increasing depth of understanding, and shedding light on those processes of a social phenomena (such as teamwork) that are difficult to narrowly define and measure, but that nonetheless play important roles in a setting. For interested readers, I have documented the details of my fieldwork and further discuss my perspective on feminist ethnography, data analysis, and academic and narrative writing processes in Appendix A.

MIXING IT UP: MULTIPLE GENRES AND CRYSTALLIZATION

One crucial aspect of ethnography is deciding how to present one's findings. Contemporary qualitative researchers engage in "creative analytic practices" that use narrative, poetic, and/or performative writing techniques to represent their findings in ways that call attention to the role of the researcher, the relationship between researchers and participants, and the ethics of speaking for others (Richardson, 2000). Such evocative accounts enable readers to experience the topic and participants in depth, rather than through reductive analysis. My goal was to provide readers as rich and nuanced an understanding of teamwork as possible. Hence, I chose to employ multiple methods of analysis and multiple genres of representation, juxtaposing social scientific academic prose with narrative representation; this mixing of genres is called *crystallization* (Richardson, 2000). The inclusion of multiple accounts enables readers not only to experience teamwork from varied angles, but also to consider the relationship between the style and content of writing.

Richardson's (2000) articulated the concept of crystallization and the capacity for writers to break out of generic constraints:

> A last evocative form to consider is *mixed genres*. The scholar draws freely on his or her productions from literary, artistic, and scientific genres, often breaking the boundaries of each of those as well. In these productions, the scholar might have different "takes" on the same topic, what I think of as a postmodernist deconstruction of triangulation . . . in postmodernist mixed-genre texts, we do not triangulate, we *crystallize*. . . . I propose that the central image for "validity" for postmodern texts is not the triangle—a rigid, fixed, two-dimensional object. Rather, the central imaginary is the crystal, which combines symmetry and substance with an infinite variety of shapes, substances, transmutations, multidimensionalities, and angles of approach . . . crystallization provides us with a deepened, complex, thoroughly partial, understanding of the topic. (Richardson, 2000, p. 934; italics in original)

Generating multiple complex understandings of the IOPOA team is my goal for this book. I included three genres—narrative ethnography, grounded theory analysis, and autoethnography (see Appendix B for a discussion of each of these methods and genres). Moreover, I explored how the three accounts represented the IOPOA team members, the patients, health communication knowledge, and me.[5] Each of the accounts was strengthened by

---

[5]My approach also was inspired by one of my feminist foremothers, Marjorie Wolf. Wolf's (1992) text, *A Thrice Told Tale*, presents an incident that occurred during her fieldwork experiences in Taiwan 30 years ago. She presents the event in the form of

my subsequent involvement in other forms of analysis; viewing my findings from different angles helped me develop a deep understanding of health care teamwork; please see Appendix C for further discussion of crystallization. The contrasting forms do not have to be thought of as conflicting. Rather they can be envisioned as complementary or as occupying points along a continuum. Multiple forms of writing "adds rigor, breadth, complexity, richness, and depth to any inquiry" (Denzin & Lincoln, 2000, p. 5). Taken together, the multiple accounts in this book illuminate the importance of backstage teamwork, its reflexive relationship with frontstage communication, and the institutional power dynamics within which both backstage and frontstage team communication occur.

OVERVIEW OF THE BOOK

Chapters 2 through 4 are ordered intentionally to provide readers with the experience of moving back and forth between contrasting styles of writing. If read sequentially, the chapters take readers through a day in the life of the clinic, analyze that daily communication through systematic categorization of communication processes, and then re-immerse readers in story, this time of my personal journey through my fieldwork, data analysis, and writing processes. However, the individual accounts are completely comprehensible when read out of order if so desired. Chapters 5 and 6, which explore power dynamics and offer conclusions, are best read after reading at least one of the accounts of teamwork (chap. 2, 3, or 4).

Chapter 2 is written as a narrative ethnography that tells a story of the team interacting in the clinical space with each other, other cancer center personnel, patients, patients' companions, and me. This is an evocative story that uses concrete details to bring readers into the IOPOA world (Ellis, 1997). I have constructed a *realistic* day in the clinic—one that resonates with verisimilitude (stays true to the essence of the clinic). I have included a variety of actual interactions that occurred during my fieldwork so that readers can glimpse the complexity of the roles enacted by the team, their patients,

---

a fictional story, a set of fieldnotes, and a scholarly article published in a mainstream anthropology journal. Additionally, Laurel Richardson's (1997) book, *Fields of Play*, features a variety of articles, essay, and poems that she has published over the last 20 years, and interspersed with "forewords" and "afterwords" that contextualize, comment on, analyze, and extend insights from the previously published pieces in the collection. Both Wolf and Richardson present multiple forms of writing in a cohesive text; I accomplish a similar goal with narrative ethnography, grounded theory analysis, autoethnography, and feminist analysis.

patients' companions, and other clinic staff. I narrate and am a character in the story, but not the main character. The narrative offers "thick description" of the communication processes that occur in the backstage, their relationship to each other, and their relationship to the team's communication with patients.

Obviously, to construct a day, I have taken liberties with chronology, condensing into a single day events that actually happened at different times during my fieldwork. I used the narrative convention of time frame (a day) to provide a sense of plot movement and improve clarity for readers. While faithfully representing the interactions I observed, I altered minor details of an interaction in service of constructing a view of the clinic that reflects the team and the people it serves in an intelligible or comprehensible manner. In addition to the chronology changes, I made two other types of changes. First, I made changes to increase comprehension for readers who are not medically trained. For example, I occasionally inserted explanations that would have been abbreviated or expressed in jargon in the team members' speech (e.g., spelled out geriatric depression scale when the social worker would have said "GDS"). Second, following Institutional Review Board ethical guidelines, I also worked extensively to protect individuals' privacy. Maintaining privacy is vital to patients and their families who generously shared their time with me during a very difficult period in their lives, and who must not be identifiable to readers. Also, I protected the privacy of team members by not including several conversations that I was asked to keep confidential or that I judged could harm the team's ability to work together if reported. To this end, I edited comments between me and team members, changed details of patients' appearance and lives, and created pseudonyms for all staff, patients, and companions. These changes made it possible to create a sense of what it feels like to spend a day with the IOPOA team in the clinic, rather than presenting a series of decontextualized (random) incidents. Ultimately, the narrative provides a comprehensible and holistic view of the IOPOA.

A grounded theory analysis of team members' backstage communicative practices forms chapter 3. This chapter provides a more analytic, social-scientific view of the clinic. Seven inductively derived categories describe the communication involved in backstage teamwork in the clinic: informal impression and information sharing, checking clinic progress, relationship building, space management, training students, handling interruptions, and formal reporting. The centrality of backstage communication to caring for patients is explored, and a view of embedded teamwork is proposed, extending on the bona fide group construct. The study provides a valuable complement to controlled studies of group decision making through its focus on dynamic communication outside of meetings among dyads and triads of team members in a weblike organization. I suggest that theorizing of communication within health care settings must take into account more thoroughly the reflexive relationship between backstage and frontstage communication and how power and privilege operate through this relationship.

Chapter 4 is an embodied autoethnographic account of my journey in the clinic (Ellis, 1997). The narrative plot reflects my process of getting to know the team and discovering/ constructing the importance to the team functioning of communication processes in the backstage area. I am the main character of this story, and it addresses my particular standpoint. This is an "embodied" tale (Denzin, 1997): My aching knee forms the background of most of my memories of that space, as does my sense of always being physically in the way of someone. In this chapter, my role as writer and interpreter is highlighted, scrutinized, celebrated, and problematized openly. Readers' understanding of the team and its communication will be heavily influenced by their understanding of who I am.

Chapter 5 offers an analysis of how power is represented and obscured in the previous three chapters. I discuss how power is manifested in embedded teamwork and in communication between team members and patients (and patients' companions). I then explore how the different modes of writing I chose to use in this book both resist and reinforce the power dynamics in the clinic that I have described and questioned.

In chapter 6, I return to the three claims about health care teams set forth in the beginning of the introduction—the crucial role of backstage communication in teamwork, the permeability of boundaries between frontstage and backstage in clinics, and the complex manifestations of institutional power and hierarchy on team communication—and explore their implications for research and theorizing of health care teamwork.

In Appendix A, I provide more extensive details of my data collection, including fieldwork, audiotaping of team member-patient interactions, and team member interviews. I then turn to a further discussion of how I conceive of narrative ethnography, grounded theory analysis, and autoethnography as individual methods in Appendix B. I explore some of the opportunities and constraints of accounts generated from these methods as I explain my approach to each and the specifics of how I utilized them. Finally, Appendix C offers further discussion of how crystallization functions in the process of analyzing and writing findings, and reflects on some of the limitations inherent in this approach to conducting research.

2

A DAY IN THE LIFE
OF THE IOPOA CLINIC

The clinic is hopping when I arrive, although it is early—not yet 9 a.m. Dr. Gino Armani has not yet come across the street from the main SRCC building to the outpatient services building. Two other physicians, who share the clinic space with the Interdisciplinary Oncology Program for Older Adults (IOPOA) team on Wednesdays, are already seeing patients. Sitting at a low desk against the wall, nurse practitioner Elaine Lyndon bends over a stack of charts. Two IOPOA patients have arrived, registered, had their vital signs checked, and are waiting in small examination rooms located side by side; the third new patient is expected shortly. Ashley Breton, the team dietitian, and Joyce Fitzgerald, the social worker, look through charts at the high counter behind Elaine, carefully making notes on their forms in preparation for seeing the patients. As I enter and call out a friendly "Hi!" to the assembled group, Elaine takes a break from her paperwork long enough to wave and flash me a smile. The doctors do not look up, but Ashley and Joyce respond with warm "Hellos."

Their heads close together, clinical pharmacist Susan Ford shows pictures of her young sons to Beth Young, the registered nurse on the team who works with Dr. Armani's patients. "Good morning," I say, leaning in to get a glimpse. The little blond boys are adorable, and I say so.

"Well, thanks," says Susan, laughing. "I like to think so!" I smile at her obvious pride in her children.

Shaking her blond head and looking thoughtful, Beth says, "They are getting so big. I can't believe my baby is now seven." Many of the women in the clinic are mothers. Three former team members went through much-discussed pregnancies while working in the IOPOA program. Pictures of babies and small children frequently find their way out of lab coat pockets and into the light to appreciative audiences. Dr. Armani has one son in college and seems to like to hear about the team members' children.

Smiling broadly, Dr. Armani comes through the doorway and approaches Beth and me as Susan walks away. "So good to see you," he says, grasping my right hand in his much larger one and placing his left hand on my forearm.

I smile at his warm greeting. "Good morning, Dr. Armani. Nice to see you."

"Good morning! Beth," he says, turning to his nurse, his broad Italian face smiling. "I have a joke for you!"

"OK," we say in unison, smiling. Dr. Armani loves to tell jokes.

"Well, the Lone Ranger rides his horse Silver out into the hills where he is captured by some Indians. They are going to kill him, but the Chief says to him, 'My people have a lot of respect for you, so we will grant you one wish before we kill you.'" Dr. Armani continues on with the slightly off-color joke. I laugh heartily at the punch line, comfortable with his fatherly persona and not offended by the crude pun, but it occurs to me that anyone who did not enjoy bantering might be reluctant to confront the director of the program over such an issue.

Beth laughs as well and then hands him a chart. "We've got six established patients for you today while you are waiting for the rest of the team to finish seeing the new patients. Mrs. Jackson is in Room 5. She has chemo today." Nodding, Dr. Armani scans the chart and turns to go down the hall to see his patient. Dr. Munson walks toward the doorway and I jump to the side, almost bumping into Elaine in my haste to make room for the man who has spoken sharply to me twice because my "chattering interferes with his ability to concentrate." I smile warily at him and he nods before turning to Laurie, the nurse practitioner who works with him.

I think back, still embarrassed, to the day when Dr. Armani and I pushed Dr. Munson too far. Only now am I beginning to see the humor in the incident. Dr. Armani loves to tease, and he and I had several go-arounds about Catholicism before this one. That morning he sauntered into the clinic at 11 a.m. because he had been on rounds in the main hospital. The always crowded space felt particularly full that morning, and Dr. Armani's patients were sharing an examination room hallway with Dr. Munson's patients. One of the computers was not working, and a young man from the information systems department was trying to fix it while Alison, an administrative assistant, leaned over him discussing the problem. A cart full of charts partially blocked the hallway, and as the nursing assistants, IOPOA team members, and Dr.

Munson's primary nurse and nurse practitioner tried to move around, we all kept bumping into each other.

"Good morning, Laura!" boomed Dr. Armani as he entered the busy desk area, mischief in his dark brown eyes.

"Good morning, Dr. Armani," I replied, smiling. I had been up late the night before working on a paper, and I was tired and my right knee ached horribly. Yet I was determined to be cheerful.

"You know, Laura," he said in his strong Italian accent, and I could see it coming. "I was thinking about all this crap you said about sex and gender and communications," he explained gleefully. "And I was thinking that the Catholic church is really the *most* feminist because of its focus on the Virgin Mary."

The former junior varsity collegiate debate champion in me bit—hook, line, and sinker. "*No way,*" I said. "The only reason they like her is that she didn't have sex. That's hardly a feminist position."

"But they elevate her above all the saints," said Dr. Armani, warming to the topic. Beth walked by, shaking her head in amusement.

"They elevate her because they are *fixated* on her virginity," I exclaimed vehemently. "They blame women for original sin, and see Mary as the only woman who somehow managed to avoid temptation. I hardly think—"

"That's not true!" shouted Dr. Armani, thoroughly enjoying my irritation. Neither of us was paying any attention to Dr. Munson, whose pale face was now red with anger. "The Virgin is valued as a woman because—"

"Would the two of you stop this!!!!" yelled Dr. Munson. I instantly cringed in humiliation, wishing the floor would open up and swallow me, but Dr. Armani just laughed. This made Dr. Munson even angrier. "You aren't even talking about a patient!! And I can't hear anything," he continued. "I can't even dictate!"

"OK, OK," said Dr. Armani soothingly to Dr. Munson. "No problem." After a last glare at my crimson face, Dr. Munson returned to his dictation. Dr. Armani turned to me and continued in a quiet voice, "We'll talk about this more later." He winked at me and patted me on the arm. I could still feel the heat in my face, and my discomfort must have been obvious to Dr. Armani because he put his arm around my shoulders and gave me a squeeze. "Don't worry." Beth approached him with a stack of prescriptions that needed his signature, and I wandered over to the opposite side of the clinic from where Dr. Munson sat, shame still coloring my face. Susan offered me a sympathetic glance and patted my shoulder as she walked by on her way to the photocopier.

Since that day, I have made it a practice to give Dr. Munson as much space as possible. Weeks later, I found out that his mother was dying in the hospital when he exploded at us that day, and he was obviously under a great deal of stress. Although he now nods at me politely and even asked once about my knee brace, I still figure that keeping my voice down and my body as far away from his as possible is the best policy.

Offering a cheery "good morning," Elaine moves past me to grab another sizable pile of paperwork that she places on a desk against the wall where she has been working. She pulls a chair up for me next to her. "You can sit over here by me," she says with a smile, well aware of my history with Dr. Munson.

"Thanks," I say, sinking down into the chair gratefully. "How are you this morning?"

"Oh, busy. We've got a full schedule today. Dr. Armani is out of town next week, so we have six established patients for him to see this morning and four this afternoon, in addition to three new patients at nine and three more at one."

I shake my head in sympathy. "Wow. They keep you on your toes!"

"Yeah," says Elaine absently, already beginning to prepare her notes for the first new patient of the morning, Mrs. Davenport. I do not want to bother Elaine, so I whip out my palmtop computer and begin jotting notes about Dr. Armani, the Lone Ranger, and my continued paranoia about Dr. Munson. I notice Beth reviewing the list of patients. The nursing assistants who bring the patients into the exam rooms and take their vital signs note on a list which patients are ready to be seen.

I smile at Beth warmly as she approaches me. "I'm about to go see Mrs. Davenport now—do my usual schpiel," she says by way of invitation. Beth prefers to orient the patients and their companions briefly on their arrival so they know what to expect during their visit, as does Jane, the nurse who works with the IOPOA's other oncologist, Dr. Josephine Klein. Depending on how busy they are, the nurses do not always get to do this, but when it happens it does seem to help avoid misunderstandings and frustration later.

"Great, I'll tag along," I say, rising from my chair. I met Mrs. Davenport and her son in the waiting room before they came in, and I am looking forward to spending some more time with Mrs. Davenport.

"Fine," says Beth, leading the way. I follow behind her slim form and wait as she knocks on the door and then opens it.

"Hi! I'm Beth, Dr. Armani's nurse," she says to Mrs. Davenport and the younger man sitting next to her. "It's nice to meet you."

Mrs. Davenport smiles. Her grayish-white skin and wig indicate that she has been having chemotherapy, but her rosy lipstick and the equally bright swaths of blusher on her cheeks give her a festive appearance. "Nice to meet you too," she says. She turns and looks deliberately at her son, who puts down the stack of papers he is reading.

"I'm Rick," he says politely. "How are you?"

Beth shakes his hand. "Fine, how are you? You've met Laura?" At their nod, she continues. "Um, today you're going to be seen by Dr. Armani. On our first visit with our patients, we do the red carpet treatment. We have a whole team of people who see you. You'll be here awhile, but we evaluate you in and out so we can get the best possible treatment plan for you. And we use a team of a dietitian, a nurse practitioner, pharmacist, social worker, and now we have Laura too."

Mrs. Davenport chuckles agreeably, her dark eyes sparkling behind her oversized brown glases. "All right," she says. Rick has returned to reading what looks like a stack of reports. He gives the appearance of a busy executive who does not like to waste time.

"So they evaluate you, give all their information to Dr. Armani, and then he'll come in an see you near the end. That way we give you something that isn't generic; we look at your whole history and make sure everything is taken care of." Beth pauses and studies Mrs. Davenport's face to see if she looks confused or concerned. She appears quite pleased, however.

Nodding, Mrs. Davenport reaches into her colorful tapestry purse and pulls out a zipper-top plastic bag containing several bottles of pills. "These are the pills I take," she says, holding the bag out to Beth. Thinking to myself that Mrs. Davenport must want to be perceived as cooperative, I smile reassuringly at her.

Beth nods. "OK. You can—"

"There are some that I only take when *absolutely* necessary," continues Mrs. Davenport.

Again, Beth nods. "Yes, you can hold on to those. The pharmacist will go through all of those with you and answer any questions you have."

"OK," says Mrs. Davenport cheerfully, placing the plastic bag on the floor by her seat.

"After everyone sees you," continues Beth, "I will come back in and make sure you don't have any other questions, and take care of anything at that time. And I'll give you my card, 'cause I'm the one you will contact if you have any questions in the future." The primary nurses are the de facto case managers, spending extensive time trouble-shooting and coordinating treatment, tests, and information flow once patients leave the new patient clinic.

Beth looks questioningly at Mrs. Davenport who nods cheerfully again. "OK, that's fine, I'll see you then," she says.

"See you then," repeats Beth, opening the door to exit.

"OK," says Rick, looking up briefly.

"I'll see you in just a bit," I say, moving to follow Beth.

"All right," says Mrs. Davenport, offering me a brief wave.

As we move down the hallway together, I ask Beth, "Isn't she sweet?"

"Yeah, she is a nice lady," replies Beth.

We pass through the doorway into the staff-only area. Beth heads to her office to check her voice mail, and I grab a momentarily vacant stool behind the left-hand counter. Susan, clinical pharmacist for the IOPOA, shakes her head as she passes through the doorway, her long muscular legs moving in quick, steady strides and her white coat billowing behind her. Casting her eyes about, she spies Ashley, the team dietitian, flipping through a patient's chart at the counter to her right, and she moves quickly to join her. I remain on my perch on a high stool behind the counter, grateful to be off my feet for a few minutes, but poised to move if any of the doctors look like they might want to use the phone in front of me to dictate about a patient.

"Hey," says Susan, catching Ashley's eye. "Great dress."

"Hi! Thanks—I went on a shopping spree last weekend." She opens her white lab coat further and tosses her long brown hair over her shoulder so Susan can get a good look. "I bought two of these dresses in different flow-ered prints, both long but with short sleeves, very comfortable," says Ashley. The yellow dress goes well with Ashley's creamy complexion.

Susan nods but then shakes her head, her brow furrowed with concern. "Have you seen Mr. Walker yet?" she asks abruptly.

Gesturing to Mr. Walker's paperwork on the counter before her, Ashley says, "I'm just getting ready to go in now. Why?"

"He's got a real problem with his Coumadin levels; they're all over the place."

"Let me guess," says Ashley. "He's taking the Coumadin with food?"

"Excuse me," says a technician trying to work his way down the crowd-ed hall.

"Sure," reply Susan and Teresa in unison, flattening themselves against the slate blue counter as he passes.

"Yes," continues Susan, straightening up. "*And* he is eating greens, you know, some days, and then none on other days. I tried to tell him he has to keep a *consistent* intake of food rich in K, but he didn't seem to go for it." Ashley nods and sighs.

This is not an unusual problem. Many of the IOPOA patients are on blood thinners such as Coumadin because of previous strokes, heart prob-lems, or blood clots. Blood thinners are difficult to regulate, especially for people who enjoy kale, chard, collards, and other greens so common on Southern tables. These foods contain high levels of Vitamin K, which thick-ens the blood. Ashley runs a hand through her thick, shoulder-length hair and picks up her pen to make a note on her nutrition screening form. "I'll be sure to stress that he needs to take the Coumadin by itself, not with any food. That should help make absorption more consistent, even if we can't get the K intake completely under control. When did he say he was taking it?"

"With lunch," answers Susan. "I suggested midmorning or midafternoon as an alternative."

"OK. Do you know if he is a snacker or pretty much a three meal a day guy?" asks Ashley.

Susan shakes her head. "No, didn't think to ask about that."

"All right, well I'll make sure I reinforce what you've said and push him to find a time at least a couple of hours after he has eaten to take the Coumadin."

"Thanks," says Susan, squeezing Ashley's arm lightly.

Ashley smiles and heads off to Mr. Walker's examination room. "No problem. Sometimes if they hear it twice, that makes a big difference. Thanks for letting me know."

"Sure," says Susan, turning toward her office.

"Susan, can I talk to you for a moment?" calls Elaine, the nurse practitioner, sounding a little tense.

Susan stiffens slightly before turning around to face Elaine with a carefully neutral expression. "Sure. What's up?" Sliding off my stool, I wander casually over to the open space between the high counters so I can better hear Elaine and Susan's interaction. Their interactions do not always go as smoothly as those between each of them and other team members, and I am curious about how they will talk. Neither of them appears to notice me.

Elaine holds up a chemotherapy order form for an IOPOA patient who is being seen by Dr. Armani before commencing her chemotherapy regimen. "You changed this chemotherapy order?"

Susan takes the form and scans it. "Yeah. The way you wrote it would have confused the pharmacists. I just straightened it out so that it used the standard language for that protocol."

Elaine sighs and runs her hand through her cropped black hair. She looks frustrated, and I think to myself for the umpteenth time that nurse practitioners are often in the difficult position of having much more medical knowledge than registered nurses but not nearly as much as physicians board certified in oncology. A thick reference book of prescription drugs and dosages bulges from her right coat pocket and provides easy reference, but I know chemotherapy agents and dosages are not listed in it. Elaine has learned a tremendous amount about geriatric oncology, but she cannot know everything. The stress of functioning, in many ways, as the hub of the IOPOA clinic practice and research process is exhausting and often frustrating, and it seems to annoy her to be corrected. "I see," says Elaine tiredly. "How was I supposed to write it?" They move to the desk where Elaine has carefully arranged charts for the patients she is seeing today. Maria, one of the clinic administrative assistants, sits in Elaine's chair looking up a patient's surgical record for Dr. Munson on one of the few computers in the clinic area. She glances up as Elaine and Susan approach her.

"I'll be right off," she says, jumping up off the chair but still typing on the keyboard. After a series of keystrokes and mouse clicks, she signs off. "It's all yours," Maria says with a smile, heading for the printer where Beth is already waiting impatiently for a printout of another patient's blood test results. Elaine sits down and Susan leans over the petite, dark-haired woman's shoulder, explaining the appropriate dosage terminology and gesturing toward the bottom of the form.

"I'm ready to report whenever you want," interrupts Eileen, the nurse practitioner student whom Elaine is currently supervising. Unlike most of the students I have seen in the clinic who are younger than I, usually in their

early 20s, this woman was a registered nurse for many years before under-
taking a master's degree to prepare her to be a nurse practitioner. Her curly
gray hair and short, squat body give her a motherly appearance.

"Give me just a minute," says Elaine without looking up. "I'm almost
done here."

Susan finishes her explanation and heads for her office. Elaine mutters
"thanks" and watches Susan walk down the hall for a moment before turning to Eileen. Joyce, the team social worker, shuts the door of a patient room
gently and approaches me as I lean on the end of a counter. Her thick blonde
hair, tinged with bits of silver, shines attractively in the harsh fluorescent
light, but her carefully made-up face is stiff with tension.

"Laura, did you see Ms. Crenshaw?" asks Joyce, her North Carolina roots
flavoring her speech.

"Um, yeah," I say. "I went in with Ashley to see her."

"Did you think she was depressed? She didn't score high on the GDS
[Geriatric Depression Scale], but I just think she is depressed." Joyce frowns.

"I thought she might be," I replied. "She doesn't seem to be handling her
diagnosis very well, and she says her husband won't talk about it." Joyce
nods silently. A moment later, I add, "He didn't come with her today; she
came with her daughter."

Joyce shakes her head with a mixture of frustration and sadness. "Well,
I talked to her about it and told her I thought she should consider seeing a
therapist and asked whether she would take an antidepressant. She said she
is afraid of antidepressants because she thinks they are addictive."

"But you think an antidepressant might help her," I say, nodding.

With misty eyes, Joyce says, "Yes. She is such a sweet lady—I feel bad.
She seems to have had a lot happen in the last few years with her children,
and her husband having a stroke. It just seems like she takes care of everyone, but now she needs to be taken care of and there's no one to do it."

I nod sympathetically as Ashley approaches us. "Are you talking about
Ms. Crenshaw?" asks Ashley.

"Yes," answers Joyce, as I nod. "I think she is depressed."

"Oh, I think so too. She seems so nice, and she obviously is having a
hard time," Ashley says. "She told me her appetite has practically disappeared, and I talked to her about the importance of regular meals and some
strategies for increasing her caloric intake."

Looking thoughtful, Joyce says, "I think I will mention it to Elaine when
I report the scores to her. Maybe if Dr. Armani explains that we have antidepressants that aren't addictive, she'll be willing to try one. I hope so." Shaking
her head slightly as if to clear it, Joyce sits down at a computer to type her
notes on this patient. She glances toward Elaine's desk periodically, waiting
for her to return from the patient she is seeing so they can discuss Ms.
Crenshaw. I follow Susan into Ms. Crenshaw's room, curious to see what
Susan's opinion of her will be and how Joyce's words may influence her.

Susan knocks on the door, pauses for a brief moment, and then opens it. "Mrs. Crenshaw?" she asks, extending her hand as she walks toward the short thin woman with wispy gray hair who sits with her purse perched on her lap, her hands carefully folded over the handles. Her daughter sits next to her, an open magazine across her lap. As Susan and I enter the room, she closes the magazine. "I'm Susan, the pharmacist with the team. How are you today?"

"I'm all right," says Mrs. Crenshaw quietly.

Her companion smiles and says, "Hello. I'm her daughter, Katherine."

I wait, smiling, until Susan shakes hands with both women before I say, "Hi again!" to the women. Turning to Susan, I add, "I met these two ladies earlier with Ashley." Susan nods.

"Yes," says Mrs. Crenshaw. "She told us she's going to school for her Ph.D. Isn't that nice?"

I smile warmly at her. Nodding, Susan says, "It sure is. Well, the reason they send me in is to talk with you about your medications." Gesturing with the piece of white paper covered in neat handwriting that details all the patient's prescriptions and their doses, she continues, "Thank you for filling this out. Not everyone does, and it is very helpful."

"Oh, you're welcome," says Mrs. Crenshaw simply.

"Now," says Susan. "I'd like to ask you about each of these drugs and what they are for, if that's all right?" Susan is always kind and friendly with her patients, but I can see her striving to be even gentler than usual with Mrs. Crenshaw.

Mrs. Crenshaw looks tired, but gamely says, "Certainly."

They work through the list together, occasionally seeking further information or clarification of a date or other piece of information from Mrs. Crenshaw's daughter. When they have reviewed each of the five medications without detecting any problems, Susan asks casually, "Do you take anything to sleep?"

"No," says Mrs. Crenshaw. "I sleep just fine. In fact, I want to sleep a lot these days."

"You're tired a lot," says Susan with sympathy.

"Yes, I am," agrees Mrs. Crenshaw, sighing.

Susan pauses and then looks down at the paper in her lap as she asks, "Have you ever taken anything for depression?"

Mrs. Crenshaw shakes her head vigorously. "No, no. I don't want to get addicted to anything like that."

"I see. Well, there are a lot of new drugs that aren't addictive, you know." Susan glances up at Mrs. Crenshaw's tense face.

"Well," hesitates Mrs. Crenshaw. "I don't know."

"Dr. Armani can talk to you more about that later if you decide you'd like to consider one," says Susan. Transitioning smoothly, she asks, "Now, what questions do you have for me?"

"None that I can think of," says Mrs. Crenshaw.

Susan digs into her lab coat pocket. "Well, here is my card, and I want you to feel free to call me if you have any questions at all about your medications." She hands the card to Mrs. Crenshaw, who passes it to Katherine, who promptly places it in her purse.

"Thank you," says Mrs. Crenshaw.

"You're very welcome. It was nice meeting you." Susan stands up and shakes hands again with both women.

"Nice meeting you, too," says Mrs. Crenshaw politely. She is slouching slightly in her chair now, fatigue clearly reflected in her drawn face and sagging shoulders.

"Bye bye," says Susan. "Feel free to call me if you think of any questions later. I'll send the next person in."

"Thanks," says Katherine.

I turn to follow Susan out the door. "I'll see you a little later with the doctor," I say as I back out of the room.

Mrs. Crenshaw nods and gives me a small smile. Katherine waves two fingers at me.

In the hallway, Susan moves down the hall a short way before saying, "She did seem depressed."

"Yeah," I say. "She's been going through a rough time."

"Mmmmm," says Susan thoughtfully. We pass Joyce, who is about to head in to see Mrs. Davenport. "She's very sweet," says Susan to Joyce, gesturing toward the room where Mrs. Davenport waits.

"Oh good," says Joyce.

"Her son is with her; he read a newspaper the entire time I was in there," adds Susan in a near whisper.

Joyce nods. "OK, thanks."

Susan walks to the desk area to type up her notes on Mrs. Crenshaw. None of the three computers is available, so she walks down the hall to her office, which has another computer, calling to Beth, "I'll be back in a few minutes." Beth, holding the telephone receiver to one ear as she apparently waits on hold, nods in acknowledgment.

Waving to Susan, I ask Joyce as she knocks on Mrs. Davenport's door, "Can I come?"

"Sure," says Joyce, with a friendly smile.

"Hi! I'm Joyce, the social worker with the team. You're Mrs. Davenport?" asks Joyce, offering her hand.

"Yes. Hello," says Mrs. Davenport, smiling.

"Is this a family member?" asks Joyce, gesturing toward Rick, who looks up briefly from his stack of paperwork.

"Yes, this is my son, Rick," says Mrs. Davenport.

"Hi, nice to meet you, too," says Joyce. Rick nods and returns to the stack of papers in his lap.

Pulling the wheeled stool up close to Mrs. Davenport, Joyce sits down. "I need to ask you about your memory and how you are doing with your treatment, see if you have any symptoms of anxiety or depression, which is really quite common with people undergoing treatment for cancer." Joyce meets Mrs. Davenport's eyes for a moment and offers a reassuring smile.

Mrs. Davenport looks quite pleased at the attention she is receiving, and not at all restless, as some patients are when confronted with the length of the comprehensive geriatric assessment process used by the team. "That's just fine!" pipes Mrs. Davenport. I notice that her periwinkle blue eye shadow reaches her carefully pencilled-in brow lines, replacing the brows she must have lost to chemotherapy. The bright eye makeup and the vibrant blush and lipstick are almost clownishly overdone, but somehow deeply endearing in the hopefulness and good spirits that they seem to reflect.

Joyce hands Mrs. Davenport a clipboard with the Geriatric Depression Scale on it, and Mrs. Davenport begins to read and check the "yes" or "no" box for each item.

"Do you feel your life is empty? No! Do you get bored? I don't have *time* to get bored! Do you feel happy most of the time? Yup! Sure do." Mrs. Davenport continues down the list, emphatically verbalizing her responses.

"That's fine, you did great," says Joyce, taking the clip board from Mrs. Davenport. "You don't seem depressed at all."

"No, I'm not. I try to keep very active. I cook and take care of the house for my son and his family. My daughter-in-law works too, you know."

"Wow, that's a lot of responsibility," offers Joyce.

"Hmm, yes, well, I like it. Rick asked me to move in with them after my husband died a few years ago."

"Well, I am sure they are glad to have you. Now I want to ask you some questions, and some of them might seem a little silly, since you obviously get along just fine. This is a test of your memory, just to see if you have more problems than most people. We all have some problems, but this is to see if there are any major problems, you know."

"Oh! I'll do my best!" says Mrs. Davenport, still smiling.

"Can you tell me today's date?"

"June 15, 1999," says Mrs. Davenport confidently.

"Good. And what city are you in?"

"Southernport." They continue on down the list of questions. Mrs. Davenport scores very well, with only one mistake. When counting backward by sevens from 100, Mrs. Davenport correctly stated "93" and "86," but then jumped to "78" instead of "79," causing the next two numbers in the series to be off by one digit as well. I am not sure I would have done any better. After reassuring her patient that the mistake is inconsequential in light of the competency she displayed on the rest of the test, Joyce turns to a discussion of Mrs. Davenport's emotional coping with her illness.

Joyce poses a few questions about her satisfaction with her living arrangements, and then asks, "Mrs. Davenport, would you be interested in support groups for cancer patients?"

"No," says Mrs. Davenport slowly. "I don't think so. I tried a couple when my husband died, and I just think I do better by myself. I have a lot of support at home and at church. I don't think so."

"That's fine. We all have our own ways of coping, and you seem to be doing just fine," says Joyce. "Do you have any questions for me, or is there anything else I could help you with?"

"No, I think I'm just fine, thank you *very* much," says Mrs. Davenport.

"OK, well here is my card. Feel free to call me if you have any questions or need anything," says Joyce, rising from her stool.

"It was sure nice talking with you," says Mrs. Davenport.

"Yes, it was. You take care now," responds Joyce, shaking her hand.

Rick looks up and smiles slightly. "Bye now," he says.

"Good bye. I'll send the next person in," says Joyce.

"I'll see you in a bit," I say to Mrs. Davenport with a wave.

"Alrighty!" she responds as we close the door behind us. Joyce and I smile to each other as we walk down the hall.

Joyce moves to the momentarily vacant chair in front of the computer that sits on the counter to the right as she enters the desk area. Setting her notes down on the counter, she begins the sequence of mouse clicks and key strokes necessary to gain access to the centralized reporting system. She looks thoughtful as she begins to type slowly and then with increasing speed as she documents her encounter with Mrs. Davenport and her son in the "OUTPATIENT BRIEF NOTE" format. The notes typed by the pharmacist, dietitian, and social worker, along with the transcribed dictation from the nurse practitioner, are used as the basis for discussing patients at the weekly team meeting, along with the screening instruments, such as the list of drugs compiled by the pharmacist and the Geriatric Depression Scale administered by the social worker.

After a few more minutes of typing, Joyce executes the command to print and slides her chair back from the counter. After retrieving two copies from the printer, she hands one to me and then she carefully places the other one in her folder. I thank her and scan it quickly.

PT is a 78 YO WWF S/P liver biopsy. She is at SRCC for evaluation by the Interdisciplinary Oncology Program for Older Adults. Not interested in support groups or counseling. She joined a support group after her husband died but did not find it useful. "I can do better by myself." She missed 3 of 30 on the mini mental status: She was unable to count backward from 100. She scored perfectly on the Geriatric Depression Scale. Pt denied any stressors at this time, seemed relatively unconcerned about possible treatment. Writer briefly discussed psychosocial services available at SRCC and gave business card to PT for future use. Pt is well-groomed with carefully applied makeup. She emphatically answered GDS questions related to happiness. No intervention appears necessary at this time. Plan: Pt will contact writer if psychosocial concerns arise. Pt and health care team aware of and agreeable to plan.

I am surprised at the cool, concise rendering of what only moments ago was a warm and lively interaction. Returning my gaze to the note, I think of what is left out: the shared laughter, Mrs. Davenport's apparent enjoyment of the attention she received and eagerness to cooperate, her son Rick's detached reading of a stack of paperwork and lack of interest in Joyce's assessment. Timothy Diamond's statement in *Making Gray Gold*—"If it isn't charted, it didn't happen"—pops into my head, and I make a note to make sure this encounter is "charted" in my writing, with as much detail possible, to document my version of what happened.

Later, I reflect on the nature of notes and dictations and wander over to the desk where Elaine is dictating in the beige telephone receiver at a rapid rate. Periodically pausing and flipping through Mrs. Davenport's chart, Elaine systematically documents the patient's chief complaint, history of present illness, past medical history, past surgical history, GYN history, chemical history, family medical history, social history, nutritional history, allergies, medications, review of systems, results of physical examination, assessment, and plan. Elaine notes such critical facts as the December 1, 1998 biopsy of Mrs. Davenport's liver tumor, the chemotherapy agents with which she has been treated thus far, her abstinence from alcohol, her allergy to penicillin, and Dr. Armani's intent to present her case to SRCC tumor board—a group of specialists who discuss treatment options for cases that do not fit established protocols.

But I know that is not all that Elaine found, I think to myself. That is *officially* what was found, but it cannot reflect the complex story that Mrs. Davenport, her son, the team members, and I constructed. I know from conversations with team members that they notice all sorts of details about patients' appearance, affect, and relationships with their companions that do not make the cut for the impersonal official documentation. Of course I think to myself as I walk across the sunny lobby to the soda machine for a Diet Coke, my version of the story is not complete either; no single story offers The Truth. I have missed many details and focused on others because of my particular perspective. I let my mind wander over the events of the morning, and Mrs. Davenport's smiling face floats persistently in my mind's eye as I think about both her uniqueness and the necessary routinization of some aspects of her care, just as with all the patients in the program.

I return to the staff area and sip my soda, leaning against one of the high counters. Rising from her chair, Elaine turns to walk down the hallway to the break room, where a pharmaceutical representative is providing a welcomed lunch of pizza and salad. The staff rarely have time to eat much of a lunch and often munch snacks at the desks as they work. I hang back. "Aren't you going to come get some pizza?" asks Elaine.

"Well, um, I wasn't sure if—," I hedge, unsure as to whether I am invited. My status as a quasi-team member has always made me somewhat uncomfortable despite that a variety of residents, physicians, nurses, and others not on the team often drop in for a share of the complimentary spreads that drug reps lavish on the team in their weekly meetings and periodically in the clinic.

"Don't be silly. There's plenty for everyone. You're part of our team," says Elaine, beckoning me with her hand to follow her.

"Well, OK, if you think it's all right," I say happily. I am very hungry, and I would kill for a chance to sit down briefly.

Susan heard the end of our exchange. "Of course you should come," she says, and the three of us walk to the break room, following the scent of parmesan cheese and oregano that lingers in the hallway.

Ashley is already eating a slice of pizza with ricotta and fresh tomatoes when I enter the room. After helping myself to a dripping wedge of the same pizza, I grab a second can of Diet Coke and pull up a chair next to hers at the crowded table. Elaine places a couple of slices on a paper plate and leaves the room, probably to work at her desk, while Susan leans against the counter as she eats. Smiling, Ashley, the dietitian, says, "Hey Laura, I read the article you wrote about ethnography and our team. I thought it was very good."

"Well, thank you," I say through a mouthful of cheese, pleased. I had given them each a copy of the publication at the conclusion of a brief talk on health communication research I had presented to them at their annual retreat the week before (Ellingson, 1998). I had not really expected them to read it, but was eager to get feedback and a little nervous that someone might object to the images of the clinic I presented.

"I really liked it too," offers Joyce. "I read it and then gave a copy to a social worker who is a survivor of a kidney transplant. She uses an approach similar to what you described in your writing."

"Thank you," I repeat, smiling broadly. "I am so glad you liked it."

"I did, because I thought you were right about our own experiences being the starting point for understanding others' experience, and how we can offer our own stories to comfort and empathize with patients," says Joyce.

"Well, I do think that's the case," I say. Ashley had turned to the woman on the other side of her, but Joyce is still looking at me, so I continue. "I have heard you all use wonderful examples about your own and your family's lives in your explanations to patients or in your efforts to offer comfort to them when they are upset."

Joyce nods, then reaches for her persistently beeping pager. Pressing a button, Joyce reads the phone number on the miniature screen, then sighs, and gets up to return the call. I smile at her and then notice that Jane, Dr.

Klein's primary nurse, is also sitting at the long table, engaged in conversation with a woman I do not know. Her short, no-nonsense gray hair and quiet nature remind me of my mother. Jane works with other physicians on days when Dr. Klein is not seeing patients in the clinic, and I suppose she is doing that again today. I have spent much less time with Dr. Klein simply because her clinic is on Tuesday mornings, and I teach on Tuesdays and Thursdays at the university, making it impossible to attend most of her clinic. She sees about a third of the IOPOA's patients, with Dr. Armani seeing the majority of the program's patients on Wednesdays. In addition to seeing patients, Dr. Klein plays an important role as the coordinator of many research studies that involve the team's patients, including a large grant application to the NIH that she and Dr. Armani have been working on for some time. She also has a well-established practice, unrelated to the IOPOA, within the cancer center.

I smile, remembering one of the days last summer that I spent in Dr. Klein's clinic. That particular morning, I arrived a few minutes before 9 a.m., my back damp with sweat from crossing the cancer center parking lot from the distant parking space I had found. The blast of the air conditioner as I entered the building was intense after the 90% humidity and the rapidly rising temperature outside that the DJs on 95.7FM had informed me was already at 87 degrees, despite the early hour of the day. I walked across the sunny lobby, now accustomed to the huge room full of patients, family, and friends who sat waiting for blood tests, chemotherapy, or an appointment with an oncologist. There must have been 30 people scattered about this morning, and quite a few of them had the bald or near-bald head topped with a scarf or baseball cap that usually accompanies chemotherapy. Many others probably were wearing wigs. Too many of them had the grayish pallor that often comes with prolonged cancer treatment.

I said hello to Ginger, the friendly, efficient woman who handles the check-in process for clinic patients. I spent one morning sitting with her and observing her and a co-worker as they processed a startling amount of paperwork necessitated by the advent of managed care and the complexity of insurance billing systems. Ginger usually wears comfortable dresses or skirts with colorful patterns that fall easily over her plump middle-aged figure, and today was no exception. Her light blue blouse contrasted pleasantly with her steel gray hair and matched the colors in her flowered skirt. She waved and smiled as she continued to process paperwork for a patient, and I passed through the door behind her desk that led from the lobby to the examination room hall. I continued on to the staff area of the clinic beyond the busy hall where two nursing assistants escorted patients into rooms.

Jane greeted me as I entered the desk area. "Good morning," she said quietly, walking deliberately but not hurriedly down the hall with the ever-present stack of paperwork resting in the crook of her right arm.

"Good morning, Jane," I responded, smiling as she continued past me and through a narrow door that led to a room full of tiny office cubicles where she had her desk. Dr. Klein came sauntering down the hall next, her sturdy body clothed in simple brown slacks and a white blouse with a small floral pattern. Her naturally curly brown hair was in its characteristic state of slight disarray. As always, the pockets of her white lab coat bulged with pens, pads of paper with trademarks of various drugs emblazoned on them, pocket reference books, notes, and a small ruler. This doctor always radiates an ease with herself and has a way of making others comfortable too. Her calm nature contrasts sharply with the effervescent, often frenetic Dr. Armani, although both of their styles are appealing and effective.

"Hello there, Laura!" Dr. Klein said brightly in her thick Swiss accent. I love the way my name sounds when she says it.

"Hello, Dr. Klein. How are you this morning?" I asked warmly.

"Fine, fine," replied Dr. Klein. "How are you?"

"Doing well, thanks," I said. I paused to see if she moved off, not wanting to take up her time if she was busy, but she stopped walking and stood with her hands clasped in front of her.

"How is your research coming?" asked Dr. Klein, looking me in the eyes to convey her sincere interest in my answer.

Flattered, I said, "Oh, it's coming along, thanks. I'm getting lots of data. I am so glad I can come to *your* clinic now that school is over for the summer, and I am not teaching on Tuesdays anymore." I watched her face carefully for her response, having always worried that she may have felt insulted by my spending the vast majority of my clinic time in Dr. Armani's clinic.

"Well, that's good," she said, no trace of irritation or defensiveness in her voice. I relaxed a little; I thought of trying to elaborate on my qualitative study, but did not know quite how to explain it. Dr. Klein has always been friendly and supportive of my presence, but at the same time she seems firmly ensconced in her positivist model of research and seems doubtful about the efficacy of my rather messy-looking methodology.

"Yeah," I agreed. "I'm looking forward to making some progress and moving on to the writing stage of the project." As I stood contemplating how to explain my multi-epistemological writing approach to a physician, Jane reappeared and said, "Josephine, can I get your signature on this order?" Dr. Klein smiled at me and then turned to Jane, taking the offered folder and reading through its contents. As I stowed my purse in a half empty cabinet beneath one of the high counters, I debated whether I was disappointed or relieved to have had our conversation interrupted before I could really attempt to bridge our different perspectives.

That morning in Dr. Klein's clinic went by quickly. I went in to see Ms. Ada Buchman with Patricia Baker, the social worker who was filling in for vacationing Joyce. It amazed me how easily Patricia slipped into the routine with the team. She carried out the same tasks as Joyce and was treated cordially by the rest of the team.

Ms. Buchman was a tiny, soft spoken woman with short white hair and pale skin. She was accompanied to the clinic today by Tony Paglio, a huge, gentle Italian-American man whose voice sounded as if he had retired to the South from the borough of Brooklyn last week instead of more than 10 years ago. Ms. Buchman sought a second opinion for a gastric cancer of unknown origin that had metastasized to her liver.

"I'm Patricia Baker, one of the social workers with the team," said Patricia, shaking Ms. Buchman's hand.

"Nice to meet you," said Ms. Buchman.

"Nice to meet you," echoed Mr. Paglio, shaking Patricia's hand as well. "I'm Tony Paglio, her, ah, friend. I take care of her." I smiled at this explanation. So many of the older folks who retire to the South are widowed or become so, and it is common for them to form new relationships with other members of their retirement communities. It appears equally common for these partnerships not to be legal marriages. I have often wondered whether this is financially motivated (the partner with the smaller social security check, usually the woman, would lose part of her income upon marriage because of the oddities of the social security system), related to concerns over wills and family inheritances, or there is a sense that marriage is not necessary because they are past the point of raising a family. There must be a myriad of reasons, and the issue intrigues me.

"Do you live together?" asked Patricia.

"Yes, we share a house over in Twin Palms, a retirement community," said Mr. Paglio. "I do all the cooking!" he added enthusiastically.

"That's wonderful," replied Patricia. Patricia smoothly transitioned into administering the Geriatric Depression Scale and then to the cognitive functioning assessment.

After we left the room together, I asked Patricia how she felt about working with the IOPOA team occasionally.

"I like it," she said simply. "It's a little different from my usual routine."

I started to ask her more questions, but Elaine interjected. "Do you have numbers for Ms. Buchman?" she asked Patricia.

"Oh, give me just a moment to calculate them," said Patricia, smiling at me apologetically as she headed for a vacant desk.

Smiling, Elaine asked, "How are you doing?"

"Oh, pretty good, thanks. How about you?" Elaine walked over to Patricia to see if she was finished with her calculations. I walked down the hall to the bathroom. By the time I returned, Elaine was finishing her report to Dr. Klein on Ms. Buchman. As they turned toward the examination room hall, I fell into step behind them. Dr. Klein smiled at me as she knocked on the door of Room 3.

"Hello!" said Dr. Klein as she entered the room where Ms. Buchman and Mr. Paglio were waiting. "I'm Dr. Klein." She shook hands with the patient and her companion.

"Nice to meet you," said Ms. Buchman quietly.

"Nice to meet you. I'm Tony Paglio, her friend," said Mr. Paglio.

Dr. Klein nodded. "OK, good. I hope things have been going well for you this morning. So how are you feeling right now?"

Ms. Buchman said unconvincingly, "Pretty good." Her small body sagged with fatigue, and her face reflected a sense of weariness and frustration.

Dr. Klein echoed, "Pretty good. Ah."

Tony Paglio jumped in, concern in his face. "She runs a fever in the evenings, at night. I called the other doctor at 1:30 in the morning, he sent us to the ER. And another time it was 102, her fever I mean. They gave her Motrin. The main thing is she feels good like she says, but she's really weak. She can't walk around the block. And she keeps getting these fevers." The words flowed forth in a rush, as if he could not wait to get them out, or perhaps he feared being cut off.

Dr. Klein nodded, turning her head to look at both Ms. Buchman and her companion. Elaine piped in, "You were anemic too, that will make you feel weak." Ms. Buchman nodded.

Dr. Klein continued, "OK. Well, the important issue is what to do now. It looks like the tumor is in your liver, metastasized to your liver, with unknown primary. But probably it began in your pancreas. You have been treated with Gemcidabene; that is the one I would choose too. So you've had some chemotherapy, and after some more, we should repeat the CT scans to see if the tumor has shrunk at all. That would be a sign that the chemo is working." She paused and looked from Ms. Buchman to Mr. Paglio and then back again, searching their faces for understanding or signs of confusion. They continued to look at her expectantly, but remained silent, so she continued. "If it doesn't seem to be working, we have some options. There are some other drugs we can try."

Ms. Buchman stared at her folded hands. Her companion spoke up, his voice tentative. "So this could be good. In other words, this thing could be clearing up." He looked torn between hope and fear.

"It could be, yes. It could be," said Dr. Klein with a slight shrug. "We won't know yet, not until we repeat the scans."

Mr. Paglio went on. "Now the object of the, the object of the treatment is to shrink the tumor around the pancreas? Or the liver?"

"It would be the same way everywhere. Ah, the tumor appears to have begun in the pancreas and spread to the liver," explained Dr. Klein patiently.

Mr. Paglio nodded vigorously. "Right." Ms. Buchman remained silent.

"And so we are certain that if the liver tumors shrink, the tumors shrink everywhere, wherever else they may be," continued Dr. Klein.

"And we will find out after several, how do I say, several treatments?" asked Mr. Paglio. At Dr. Klein's nod, he continued. "She took a blood test yesterday, and she has one more tomorrow."

"OK," said Dr. Klein, waiting to see where this is leading.

Mr. Paglio said, "We will know, in other words, from the test."

Dr. Klein looked mildly perplexed and tried again to explain. "Your oncologist continues the treatment, as he does now. Then she will come back and um, usually we do blood tests every month or so. The CT scan, I only do that every 2 months. It takes that long for there to be any change in the tumor size that would show up on a CT scan, if the chemo is working. So it doesn't make sense to do it more often than that." Dr. Klein peered directly into Mr. Paglio's eyes, gauging his comprehension. Ms. Buchman remained silent, looking more and more tired.

Mr. Paglio shook his head and countered with some urgency, "But when they gave us the three treatments of the chemo, the girl made *sure* that she went straight to check her blood." As he says "her blood," he touches Ms. Buchman gently on the arm with his huge palm. It piques my interests as I lean against the counter in my usual spot that Mr. Paglio had said, "us" rather than "her." It is clear that the treatment of his partner is very upsetting to him.

"Ah, right," said Dr. Klein.

"And that same day was either Monday or Tuesday before her Wednesday treatment," said Mr. Paglio, as if that explained everything.

Still not sure what he was getting at, Dr. Klein said, "OK," and nodded encouragingly for him to continue.

Mr. Paglio said, "Now is that some sort of, ah, that would be some sort of an evaluation?" He looked at the doctor hopefully.

Dr. Klein shook her head, understanding that he was asking if the blood test would reveal whether the chemo was working. "It's an evaluation," explained Dr. Klein. "But it is looking at white blood cell count. You need to check the blood each week to make sure you are well enough to have another chemotherapy treatment. If Ms. Buchman does not have enough white cells, that needs to be treated. We have a drug called Neupogen that makes the body grow white cells. That is why she keeps getting those fevers. They are called neutropenic fevers, because she doesn't have enough white cells in her blood. Those tests don't tell us whether the chemo is shrinking the tumor or not."

Mr. Paglio nodded his understanding, his face reflecting his disappointment with her explanation. It was clear he wanted to know if these drugs that were rendering his loved one so weak were helping her. After a moment, he said thoughtfully, "Now about the pancreas. There is just, I understand that, when they take x-rays of the pancreas they just can't see everything they want to see. But when you look at these slides or whatever you look at these x-rays do you see it in the pancreas or on or around the pancreas."

Dr. Klein asked, "Do you want to look at the scans while we talk about this? I'll go get them." She jumped up from her stool and headed out the door without waiting for an answer. Elaine and I stayed with the patient and her companion.

Elaine said, "OK. So, I wouldn't worry about that one around the pancreas; because you have to wait a little more to get more chemo before you can make a judgment."

Mr. Paglio said, "The only reason I say that is, ah, when we went to Dr. Charett, he had said we don't see nothing in the pancreas."

"That's right," said Elaine.

"The only thing we see is a haze," said Mr. Paglio.

"Right," repeated Elaine.

Aware that he was not making himself understood, Mr. Paglio tried again. "You know what I'm saying? In other words they're treating her for the pancreas, is that correct?"

Elaine shook her head. "No, they're treating her for the liver."

"Oh, it's the liver," said Mr. Paglio with surprise.

Elaine continued, "Her only proof of disease is in the liver. That's the only place she had a biopsy."

Mr. Paglio responded, "But they don't know any other place where they believe it's coming."

"Right. And there might be some in the pancreas, but it doesn't matter as long as she gets her treatment, and she responds in the liver, that'll be good enough. And if she doesn't respond in the liver then we need to change her to something else."

"I see," said Mr. Paglio in a tone that did not resonate with his words.

Elaine sensed at least some of his hesitation. "Got it?" she asked.

Mr. Paglio shakes his head. "You know, because they were saying, from what we understood, we have to find out where it's coming from."

Dr. Klein walked back in the room. Elaine said to her, "He's worried about the pancreas because he was told that the liver mass came probably from the pancreas."

Dr. Klein nodded and removed three CT scan films from a large brown envelope. She slid a lighted board out from what I had thought was a drawer in the counter, and placed one of the films on it. "Here we are. OK. I need to find one where we will be able to see." She took out a pile of CT scan films and flipped through the dates and different views until she found one she liked. This one she laid on the lighted board in front of her. Picking a pen from the assortment in her pocket, Dr. Klein used it to point to various places on the scan. "You see that here is where the cancer is in your liver. The gray spot here. They are not very big, actually. You have several of them."

Ms. Buchman leaned over to inspect the scan and said with some excitement, "Liver! That's the liver!" I was glad to see her contributing to the conversation.

Dr. Klein nodded. "That's the liver and um you have this big thing here is the liver and the liver as you know can really function with only 1/10th of its cells and still function very well. OK. Now the pancreas is a little more difficult to see, but it's a little large here and that's why we are kind of suspecting, you know, that it started from here."

Elaine added, "But we can give your treatment while following the liver because it's easy to see." She paused and searched Mr. Paglio's face for comprehension. "Are you clear, Mr. Paglio?"

"I'm clear," he said unconvincingly. "I wasn't . . . " His speech trailed off, and he looked confused and tentative.

Dr. Klein looked concerned. "Did I misunderstand what you were asking?"

Mr. Paglio shook his head. "No, you explained it very well. We didn't understand that. You see what happened was the physician before you said that he sees in the liver two lumps, and they said they believe it came from the pancreas, and you can't x-ray the pancreas as well as they'd like to. But they see a little haze or whatever they call it. So, the way I understood it, they were going to treat the pancreas, and the whole thing would clear up or stabilize. Er, so that's the way we understood it, but I thought they weren't sure about that."

Dr. Klein nodded emphatically. "It's not 100% sure. The pancreas is an organ that the cancer usually cannot be seen in. Often all you see is the pancreas getting larger than it should. But the treatment should help *both* the liver and the pancreas." She pauses and looks from Ms. Buchman to Mr. Paglio before continuing. "The treatment is the same, we just watch the tumor in the liver because we can see it well. If it didn't start in the pancreas, the treatment should still help wherever it started from, whatever that organ or tissue is. And we can still track that progress in the liver using the CT scans." Ms. Buchman and Mr. Paglio nodded, appearing to understand. The discussion was wrapped up quickly after that. I still wasn't confident that Ms. Buchman and Mr. Paglio understood the rational behind her treatment plan, but they appeared happier and more relaxed.

I reflect back on that day in Dr. Klein's clinic as I continue to eat my lunch. After I finish another delicious slice of pizza, I throw away my paper plate and napkin, and take one last swig of my Diet Coke before tossing the can in the trash. It occurs to me that this treat would be a great addition to the daily clinic work.

As I make my way back to the desk area, I frown, thinking of Ms. Buchman and how difficult it often is to explain confusing and counter-intuitive information about cancer treatment to people who do not have medical training. Despite having been through cancer myself and having observed an oncology team for almost 2 years, I still miss a lot of what the team members discuss. There are so many drugs, tests, and symptoms that it is difficult to keep all of the terminology straight. My heart goes out to the patients and their loved ones as they try to grasp the technical information while coping with the emotional pain that accompanies a cancer diagnosis.

I brace myself for another set of patients as the little hand on the clock nears the one position. Sheri, the nursing assistant in the clinic today, has brought back the first of the afternoon patients and marks that on the list taped to the bedside table that remains in the desk area for the sole purpose of holding that list. She waves to me, smiling, and then returns to the waiting room to see if others have arrived. Sheri is always friendly to me, but I do not often see her talking with other team members, except when they are asking her which patients are ready to be seen. Perhaps this is simply because I have more time available for chatting than the team members.

Twenty minutes later, Susan closes the door to a patient's room and strides into the desk area. Turning, Joyce and Ashley say in unison, "Who did you see?" and then laugh at their accidental coordination.

"Ms. Tuttle," responds Susan cheerfully. A beeper sounds its shrill tone, and everyone in the immediate vicinity looks down to see if it is theirs. I used to find it mildly amusing the way the entire group would simultaneously glance at their waist bands at the sound, but now I am as used to it as they are and do not pay much attention.

This time it is Ashley's, and she lays her folders on the counter and reaches for the phone. After a quick discussion and a glance at her watch, she returns to her paperwork, sighing. "The breast cancer program wants me to come see a patient across the street. But I have to finish up here first." Ashley looks mildly annoyed. She is very conscientious and hates to keep a patient waiting, but she can only be in one place at a time. Grabbing the paperwork, she hurries down the hall to her next patient.

"Would you mind if I tagged along?" I ask Ashley, as she heads for Mrs. Antonucci's examination room to conduct a dietary assessment.

"Not at all," replies Ashley with a smile. I fall into step beside her as we approach Room 5.

Ashley knocks and enters, "Mrs. Antonucci? I'm Ashley, the dietitian."

"Nice to meet you," says Mrs. Antonucci quietly. Her hair is carefully coifed, and she wears crisp blue pants and a white cotton blouse.

"And you must be . . .?" Ashley diplomatically leaves the question hanging as she offers her hand to the gentleman sitting to Mrs. Antonucci's left. I smile to myself, having seen the humorous and not-so-humorous reactions when team members guess incorrectly about a companion's identity, addressing a wife as a daughter or a brother as a husband.

"Dominic Antonucci, her husband," he says gruffly, shaking her hand. Mr. Antonucci and his wife are both short, hardly over 5 feet, and their weathered faces reflect their Italian heritage.

"Nice to meet you too," says Ashley. Turning toward me, she steps back so I can shake their hands too.

"I'm Laura Ellingson. It's nice to meet you. I am a Ph.D. student in the Communication Department. I am studying how the staff members communicate with patients today, and I'd like to observe while you talk with Ashley, if that is OK with you?" I look questioningly at Mrs. Antonucci, who looks down.

"Well, that's all right, I guess," says Mr. Antonucci. I try to catch Mrs. Antonucci's eye for her approval, but she does not look up.

"Okay, thank you," I reply brightly, leaning against the counter as Ashley pulls the short rolling stool up close to Mrs. Antonucci.

Ashley looks directly at Mrs. Antonucci. "OK, I need to ask you a few questions about your eating habits, and then depending on how you answer those, I might have a few more. Then I will take a couple of simple measurements, and we'll be done, OK?"

"That sounds—" begins Mrs. Antonucci, before her husband cuts her off.

"When are we going to see the doctor?" interrupts Mr. Antonucci, irritation evident in his voice.

"You will see the doctor after you see me and the rest of the team. Who have you seen already?" asks Ashley calmly.

"We saw a pharmacist and a nurse," replies Mr. Antonucci. Mrs. Antonucci nods.

"Well," says Ashley, looking at Mrs. Antonucci, "after I talk with you, you will also see a social worker and a nurse practitioner. We all gather information that we pass along to the doctor so he can make the best decision about your wife's care." Ashley turns and gazes intently at Mr. Antonucci, whose tightly pressed lips signal his annoyance, but who declines to comment.

Ashley turns back to Mrs. Antonucci. "I'd like to get a sense of what you eat on a typical day. What do you usually eat for breakfast?"

"I—" says Mrs. Antonucci.

"Well," interrupts Mr. Antonucci. "I have some eggs or corn flakes."

Ashley's expression remains carefully neutral. "Um-hmm. Is that what you usually eat as well, Mrs. Antonucci?" The patient nods silently. Mr. Antonucci glares at Ashley. "OK, and about how many glasses of water would you say you drink per day?"

Mr. Antonucci answers quickly, "She drinks at least three or four." Mrs. Antonucci looks at her wrinkled hands.

Struggling to keep the anger I feel toward Mr. Antonucci off my face, I wonder whether Ashley is having to work at remaining pleasant as well. As the interview continues, Mr. Antonucci continues to answer all questions directed at his wife while Mrs. Antonucci slumps in her chair tiredly. The older woman looks exasperated, but whether with her husband, Ashley, or the length of the visit in general is unclear. Ashley continues to address her questions to her patient, making eye contact with Mrs. Antonucci whenever the older woman looks up from her lap. After measuring Mrs. Antonucci's right upper arm and right calf, Ashley smiles at both of them and says, "That's all I need. Do you have any questions for me?"

Mr. Antonucci immediately and firmly says, "No." Mrs. Antonucci shakes her head.

"All right, well it was nice to meet you. Here—"

"OK, yeah," says Mr. Antonucci impatiently.

Ashley continues, "—is my card. Feel free to call me if you have any questions for me later. Bye."

"OK," say Mr. and Mrs. Antonucci together.

"It was nice to meet you," I say, backing out of the room. Mrs. Antonucci nods; Mr. Antonucci looks down at the appointment card clasped in his hand.

Out in the hall, Ashley rolls her eyes.

"If my husband ever treated me like that . . . ," I say quietly, but vehemently.

"I know," replies Ashley with a nod. Her long brown hair falls over her shoulder, and she pushes it back absently. "Me too." Approaching the desk area, we see Susan typing a note on one of the computers. I hesitate, curious as to what, if anything, Ashley will say to Susan. "Hey—we just saw the Antonuccis," says Ashley.

Susan rolls her eyes as she says, "He didn't let her say a word while I was in there. He wouldn't even let me look at the medication list; he *insisted* on reading it to me."

"Well, he did the same thing with Ashley," I interject. "It drove me crazy."

"It was pretty bad," says Ashley.

"Maybe we should tell Joyce before she goes in," I offer casually, uncertain of whether I should be meddling, but concerned about Mrs. Antonucci.

"Yeah," says Susan, nodding. "Let's tell her, and we better warn Elaine too." Joyce emerges at that moment from one examination room and, glancing down at her folder of paperwork, heads across the hall to her next patient. "Joyce!" calls Susan, jumping up from her seat.

Walking to the doorway that separates the examinations rooms from the staff desk area, Joyce leans her small frame against the frame. "Yes?" she asks. Susan approaches her, glancing at the room where the Antonuccis wait to ensure that the door is closed before she continues. Quietly, she explains the situation to Joyce and suggests that she try to see Mrs. Antonucci alone.

Joyce nods. "That sounds like a good idea. I will tell him that it is our policy to do psychosocial assessments with the patient alone." Joyce pauses and looks thoughtful. "It would be nice if we had an errand for him to run or something. Some reason to get him out of there. I've got one more patient to see before them." Joyce returns to the examination room hall, and Beth enters the desk area as I furiously jot notes.

Beth declares to no one in general, "The Antonuccis are threatening to leave in 10 minutes if they don't see Dr. Armani by then. They've been here since quarter of one, and it's almost three now." She says this matter of factly. Elaine nods, but does not look up from her perusal of files on her desk. I wonder whether she heard Beth's comments over the din produced by one ringing phone, Dr. Munson talking on another phone, and Dr. Zertan having a heated exchange on yet another phone.

"Elaine, perhaps you should go in there and do damage control," suggests Susan casually. "He is really angry, and he would hardly let his wife speak to either me or Ashley."

Sighing as she stands up, Elaine says, "Ugh. Well, OK."

"Good luck," I offer sympathetically. Not wanting to get in the way of her efforts to soothe the angry couple, I don't ask to tag along, but I am dying of curiosity about how she will handle Mr. Antonucci.

"Well," says Elaine. "Sometimes this works and other times it doesn't." Shaking her head as if to clear it, Elaine walks quickly to the Antonuccis' examination room. She is gone less than 5 minutes and returns smiling. "He's difficult, but thank God they're Italian and from Long Island. I'm from Long Island, so we talked about that and I promised to have Armani in there soon. We joked about cannolis." Shifting gears smoothly, Elaine returns to the report she is preparing. I stare in amazement and then jot some more notes. The incident makes me think of Sandra, the nurse practitioner who was with the team from its inception through my first year of fieldwork. She was good at diffusing anger with patients as well, but what really struck me was how well she responded to distraught patients.

I remember one day I arrived and Sandra was perched on a stool behind one of the high counters, pouring over a chart and making notes on her intake form.

"Hi, Sandra!" I said as I walked into the desk area.

Sandra looked up and smiled her huge, warm, light-up-her-face smile. "Good morning, Laura! I am so glad you're here today."

"Thanks," I said happily, stowing my purse underneath the counter in one of the cabinets. "How are things going?"

"Busy," said Sandra simply, returning to her paperwork.

Ellen Darren, the dietitian who preceded Ashley, came into the desk area and walked over to Sandra. "Hi Laura," she said to me. "How are you?"

"Fine, thanks," I replied. "How are you?"

"Fine, thanks," said Ellen. Turning to face Sandra, she continued, "Sandra, I just saw Ms. Viola. She is very sweet and very articulate. She is an artist, very interesting, and has an excellent diet. Not at risk. I'll have her BMI number for you in a minute."

Sandra listened attentively and nodded. "Great."

"She only has Medicare and lives on Social Security, so I'm not sure how she ended up here," wondered Ellen. "She got a referral from another doctor, I think, but still . . . " She shrugged and let her voice trail off. What she did not say is that the vast majority of the patients in the senior program, indeed in the whole cancer center, have good quality insurance and/or a good Medicare supplement and middle- or upper class incomes. That results in a predominantly White clientele because people of color are overrepresented among the poor. I thought to myself that the patients at the public hospital are not likely to get the careful screening they get here because of all the staff and time a comprehensive geriatric assessment requires. The team here generally reaches a fairly elite group of patients.

Sandra nodded, understanding Ellen's meaning. "Thanks. I'm heading in to see her now," she said. Turning to me, she asked, "You coming?"

"Sure, thanks," I said, following her tall slim figure down the hall.

Sandra knocked on Ms. Viola's door and then entered with me right on her heels. "Ms. Viola?" inquired Sandra. At the petite, white-haired woman's nod, Sandra introduced herself. "Hi! I'm Sandra Bates, the nurse practitioner with the program. I'm so glad you've come to see us today." Sandra shook hands with her patient and then gestured toward me. "And this is Laura," she said.

"Hi!" I said, "I'm Laura Ellingson, and I'm in the Ph.D. program in Communication. I'd like to watch how the staff communicates with you today, if that's all right." The words, spoken dozens of times, spill out of my mouth effortlessly, but as always, I carefully watch for the patient's reaction so I can excuse myself and leave if she seems uncomfortable with my presence. Most patients respond quite enthusiastically, often asking me questions about my research. Only once or twice has a patient looked so uncomfortable that I left.

"That's fine with me," said Ms. Viola. "You're studying communication?"

"Yes," I answered. "I am trying to understand how doctors and nurses and others communicate with patients."

"All right," she said, nodding.

"Thank you," I said, moving to lean against the counter. I noted her neat cotton blouse, cardigan sweater, and white "pedal pushers," as my grandmother calls them. I also noted that she had come to her appointment alone, which was unusual. Most patients bring at least one companion, and quite a few bring two or even three.

Sandra smiled at me and then drew her stool up close to Ms. Viola. "The records they sent us aren't very complete, so I want to go over your medical history with you and fill in a few holes."

Ms. Viola nodded patiently. "OK," she said simply.

"Any history of heart disease?" asked Sandra.

"No."

"Stroke?"

"No."

"Diabetes?"

"No."

Sandra proceeded down the list of common ailments with Ms. Viola repeating her mantra of "no" to all of them. "Any difficulty getting around?" asked Sandra next.

As if she had been waiting for just such a question, Ms. Viola took a deep breath and began, "Yes, I do. I have fibromylagia, and it is very painful in my hands. And I am so tired, and my back aches and so does my rib cage, and I can't work." Sandra nodded, and Ms. Viola continued. "The pain is so bad I can't sit at my drawing table. I am a very creative person. That's who I am— I am a professional visual artist. If I can't do my work, I'm not *me*," she finished passionately.

Sandra nodded sympathetically, concern for Ms. Viola evident in her sad expression. "I'm so sorry. That must be very upsetting. And the pain is mostly in your back?" asked Sandra.

"My back and my ribs. I'm having trouble walking any distance now. I don't have a car, and so I have to take the bus. I live in Jackson Heights," she added, referring to a run-down area in the heart of the city. "I can't carry my groceries any more from the bus stop all the way to my apartment. I feel exhausted all the time." Leaning forward, Ms. Viola looked Sandra straight in the eyes, seeking validation.

Sandra did not disappoint her. "That's rough," she said kindly. "I can see how that would be very difficult for you. Well, we are going to do our best to figure out what is wrong with you and do everything we can to help you feel better. I'll make sure to pass along this information to Joyce, our social worker, too. She may be able to help you out with transportation."

"It is difficult. I don't have much money, and the area I live in isn't safe, you know," said Ms. Viola. "And if I have cancer, I just don't know what I will do." Ms. Viola looked like she was on the verge of tears.

Sandra continued to nod sympathetically and handed her the box of tissues from the counter. Ms. Viola took one and dabbed her eyes. "I understand," said Sandra sincerely. "Dr. Armani is probably going to need to do some more tests to determine just what may be wrong. We don't want to jump to any conclusions." Sandra reached over and squeezed Ms. Viola's hand briefly, waiting while her patient took some deep breaths and regained her composure. After a few moments, Sandra said gently, "I need to ask you a few more questions, OK?" Ms. Viola nodded. "Do you smoke?"

"Let me tell you my smoking history," said Ms. Viola. "Do you want to hear it?" she asked hopefully.

"Of course," said Sandra brightly, as if she did not have two patients waiting, numerous phone calls to return, and other patients' visits to dictate, and she wouldn't prefer just a simple yes or no answer. Sandra let her folder of paperwork sink to her lap and looked Ms. Viola straight in the eye.

Ms. Viola relaxed her tense shoulders somewhat and smiled cheerfully. "When I was in art school—I put myself through art school in Buffalo, New York—I decided it would be *very* cool to smoke," began Ms. Viola. "So I went with my girlfriend to buy a pack of cigarettes, and then we each lit one and stood there holding it. I didn't even inhale!! I thought I looked very dramatic holding it, though." She paused and looked to Sandra, who nodded encouragingly, and then she glanced my way. Smiling, I nodded for her to go on. "So I kept doing that for *weeks*, and then I finally said to myself, 'This is stupid, and I can't afford it.' I gave it up, and I haven't touched another one since!" finished Ms. Viola triumphantly.

"Good for you! What a wonderful story!" said Sandra, smiling. "We all do foolish things when we are young, don't we?"

"Yes, we sure do," replied Ms. Viola.

"OK, I need to do your physical exam now." Sandra stood up and opened one of the drawers beneath the examination table. "I'm going to give you one of our beautiful designer gowns," she joked.

"Oh, lovely," said Ms. Viola with a smile.

Sandra placed her hand lightly on Ms. Viola's forearm. "Just take off your top and bra. You can leave your slacks and underpants on, OK?"

"OK," said Ms. Viola, unbuttoning the top button of her sweater.

"We'll step out of the room now so you can change," said Sandra, moving toward the door. I followed. "See you in a couple of minutes," Sandra said reassuringly, shutting the door behind her.

When we got out into the hall, Sandra walked to the desk area, and I followed close behind her. She seemed lost in thought and did not say anything. She began sorting through some paperwork on the desk as if looking for something. Finally, I said, "She was interesting. What did you think?"

Sandra looked up at and smiled at me. "She just needed to be heard," she said quietly.

That demonstration of compassion, and now the one between Elaine and the Antonuccis, are just two of the many I have witnessed between each of the team members and their patients. I am amazed at their capacity for caring, day after day. I look up from my note-taking as Dr. Armani approaches Elaine.

"Are you ready?" asks Dr. Armani, leaning over Elaine as she flips through a stack of paper work on her crowded desk.

"Mmm, yeah, just a minute," mumbles Elaine without looking up. Dr. Armani walks away impatiently to sit at the high beige counter that runs the length of the back room of the clinic. Snatching up the phone receiver, he punches the speed dial code for the central dictation computer and proceeds to dictate on an established patient visit. When he is finished about 3 minutes later, Elaine is waiting in front of the light board with Mr. Morton's chart, CAT scans, and pathology reports. "Ready for Mr. Morton?" she asks.

Nodding, Dr. Armani walks over. "OK, go ahead."

Elaine takes a deep breath. "Mr. Morton is a 71-year-old man diagnosed with multiple myeloma in 1992. Gradual onset of paralysis in his lower back and legs led to the diagnosis. Surgery was performed to remove a tumor in the vertebrae, which was then followed up with 15 radiation treatments. He had three courses of chemo that was discontinued after a liver reaction. Then he had a 96-hour continuous drip of another chemotherapy drug, then radiation for tumors in the pelvis and femur. In February of this year, tumors were located in T5 and T6, and he began a series of seven doses of chemotherapy for those. He has had severe neutropenia and low red blood cells and was hospitalized for neutropenic fevers and cardiac problems. He says his oncologist told him that the chemo wasn't working and discontinued it, but then called him in a week later and said that blood tests show the tumors are responding. They are here for a second opinion. These are his CT scans."

"Thanks," says Dr. Armani, flicking on the light board and hanging the first of three images on it. "All right, let's go," he says after scanning all of the images briefly. A moment later, I am hurrying down the hall behind Dr. Armani, shaking my head over how fast he assimilates information and reaches decisions.

"Hello!" booms Dr. Armani as he moves his tall, broad-shouldered frame into the crowded examination room. "Mr. Morton? I'm Dr. Armani. It's so nice meeting you." Mr. Morton shakes the doctor's offered hand.

"Hello," says Mr. Morton with a smile. Mr. Morton is a short man with a big belly that gives him a faintly gnome-like appearance. Wispy tufts of white hair floated around his mostly bald head, speckled here and there with brown age spots. He wears a cotton shirt with images of golf paraphernalia pictured on it, khaki polyester pants, and brown loafers.

"You are Mrs. Morton?" asks Dr. Armani of the woman sitting next to him. She is about the same height as her husband. Blue shorts and a matching cotton shirt fall softly over her plump body. Behind glasses her eyes sparkle, and a wealth of laugh lines testify to her friendly disposition.

"Yes, hello," answers Mrs. Morton, smiling broadly as they shake hands.

Mr. Morton gestures toward the younger woman to his left. "And this is my daughter, Melanie."

Dr. Armani shakes the young woman's hand vigorously. "Nice meeting you, too. So glad you could come." The Morton's daughter appears to be in her mid-30s and, like her parents, she wears casual cotton clothing suitable for the hot, sticky weather we are experiencing. Pulling a rolling stool up close to Mr. Morton, Dr. Armani places his hand on his patient's forearm and continues, enunciating carefully, "I hope you won't have that much problem with my accent. I was born and raised in Italy and still have a strong accent after living in America for 25 years."

"I'm OK," says Mr. Morton.

"Do you understand me well?" asks Dr. Armani, glancing at Mrs. Morton and their daughter.

Mr. Morton says, "Oh yes," and the women nod in agreement, their eyes wide with hope and fear and their torsos leaning slightly forward in anticipation of the doctor's words.

Dr. Armani smiles and continues, his large hand still resting lightly on Mr. Morton's arm. "Elaine tells me that you want to know what to do next, is that right?"

Mr. Morton lifts his head, straightens his shoulders, and looks Dr. Armani in the eye. "I'd like to know what my destiny is," he says quietly in a serious tone.

Dr. Armani nods and the smile leaves his face. He runs a hand through his short, thick, dark hair, which increasingly is flecked with gray. "Well, let me tell you," he begins. "I went through all of your charts, which are very complex. And it looks like the treatment that Dr. Wilson has been giving to you right now has been working. Your protein levels were very high before, and now they are down to a normal level as indicated in your blood test." Dr. Armani pauses and looks at Mrs. Morton and Melanie. They both nod in acknowledgment, and he proceeds. "So I definitely think that treatment is working. Obviously, though, there is a price to pay besides the cost of the treatment."

Mr. Morton's face is tense, and his lips are pressed together in a slight frown. "Yeah," he offers simply.

"The price is that your blood count goes down. Your hemoglobin is low, and so are your white blood cells, and ah, you are aware of that?" Dr. Armani raises his brows questioningly and again looks at the patient, his wife, and his daughter in turn. Each of them nods. "OK, ah, one thing that I've not seen in your record, but maybe Dr. Wilson has been doing. Did he ever give you some shots of ProCrit?"

Mr. Morton perks up slightly. "Periodically."

Mrs. Morton nods in agreement. "Yes," she says. "He gets those after every chemo treatment."

Dr. Armani appears pleased. "Good. That is to stimulate the production of red blood cells." Dr. Armani pauses and looks down at the floor for a moment. Raising his head and meeting Mr. Morton's eyes, he clears his throat and tightens his grip a little on Mr. Morton's arm. "And now, your disease is not a curable disease—you are aware of that?" He watches Mr. Morton's face carefully for his reaction.

"But they're working on a cure here, aren't they?" he responds evasively.

Dr. Armani sighs. "Well, we're working to see whether it's treatable in two ways. One is with the bone marrow transplant, but thank the Lord, you are not a candidate for that." Dr. Armani does not explain why the patient is not a candidate or why he is happy about that. I have heard Dr. Armani expound at team meetings about the high risk involved with bone marrow transplants. Although I have not read the medical journal articles on the topic, Dr. Armani cites numerous studies that indicate that the treatment kills far more patients than it benefits. In his opinion, this treatment is an example of the fearful public unwisely demanding insurance coverage for a treatment that has not been shown statistically to prolong life or to be effective in treating most of the types of cancer for which it is used.

Dr. Armani continues, "The other treatment is with something new. We are trying to use some new chemotherapy for multiple myeloma. But I would not change the one that you have received yet because so far it has been working." Morton's daughter jots notes quickly on her pad.

Mr. Morton is disappointed; his small shoulders slump against the back of the wooden chair he sits in, and his eyes look teary. "All right," he says with resignation, looking down at the light brown carpet.

"The question now is whether you should receive the next chemo treatment soon. Ah, when is the next one?"

Mr. Morton pauses and his wife speaks up quickly. "It's June 30th," she says confidently.

Mr. Morton nods in agreement. "Yeah, sometime in June."

"It may be wise, especially since the hemoglobin seems to have gone down, to wait awhile before the next course of treatment to give some more time to your system to recover. We'd be glad to call the doctor and talk to him about that if you want me to."

"OK, yes, thanks," says Mr. Morton.

Dr. Armani continues, "Basically I agree with everything that was done. I—"

Mrs. Morton interrupts, "Well, that's one thing we came here for. If we heard that we had done the right thing, then we'd be happy, you know." She looks at Dr. Armani anxiously.

Dr. Armani nods at the familiar sentiment. So many patients and family members are wracked with guilt, believing that if they had gone to a cancer center initially that the patient would have had better treatment and a better prognosis. This usually is not the case. Moving his gaze among the family members, he says slowly and with conviction, "We would *not* have done *anything* differently if you had come here first. Your doctor has treated you using the same protocol I would have used. There are not a lot of options for your disease." Melanie continues to scribble away on her notes as Mr. and Mrs. Morton exchange a look of profound relief. Dr. Armani straightens his shoulders and removes his hand from Mr. Morton's arm. "Now, you know," continues, "I cannot micromanage your disease from here."

Mr. Morton smiles, "Oh I understand that," he says.

Dr. Armani nods. "Good. So, basically, Dr. Wilson does excellent work and ah, the only thing I could suggest would be maybe to give you a little more time to recover from one treatment to the other. And maybe to give you some more shots to make you feel a little stronger."

"Right," says Mr. Morton. "You talking with Dr. Wilson is fine by me, you know. I'd like that." He pauses and then continues, looking at Dr. Armani intently. "I've gone through all these treatments. I just, when Dr. Wilson did that 180-degree turn, from what he told us in the hospital—that the chemo wasn't working anymore, and he said we'll stop it—well, I was crushed. Then a week later, we go to his office and come to find out a new blood test he had taken showed it looked good again, that the chemo was working after all."

Dr. Armani smiles and gently places his hand on Mr. Morton's arm again. "Those are the happy surprises that happen from time to time," he says kindly. Mr. Morton smiles, seeming both hopeful and fearful. Dr. Armani looks thoughtful and says, "I've had one of those experiences myself. A lady with cancer of the pancreas came in here 3 years ago. She was very sick. I started her on the chemotherapy, but after 2 weeks we stopped the treatment because her mouth became all covered in sores. And so I wasn't optimistic about her prognosis, but I was already talking to her about going through treatment with the experimental agent. I said, let's take another CT scan before that. And then the CT scan showed that the cancer was gone. She stop taking any chemo, and she's doing well now. Sometimes things work better than we foresee."

All of the Mortons smile with renewed hope. "All you people have to do is keep me alive until your experimental cure is completed!" chimes Mr. Morton.

Dr. Armani chuckles. "I promise that we will work on that."

Melanie speaks up for the first time since the doctor entered the room. "I have a question," she says quietly.

Dr. Armani leans away from Mr. Morton and swivels his stool toward Melanie. "Please go ahead," he says. "I did not mean to cut you off."

"No, no, that's OK, you didn't," says Melanie. "But if the last chemo treatment that he had resulted in neutropenia . . ."

Dr. Armani nods. "Neutropenia, yes."

Melanie asks intently, "What are the chances of that happening again?"

"Unless something is done, one hundred percent." Seeing the crestfallen faces of the Mortons, Dr. Armani quickly adds, "OK, so there are two or three ways this can be handled. One is to decrease the dose of chemotherapy. That's a possibility. Two is to have Neupogen shots after the chemotherapy. That's a shot to stimulate the production of white blood cells. The other is to give him some medications that contain steroids. But I'm sure Dr. Wilson will take care of that. I cannot speak for him, but anyway we will talk about this with him. Any other questions?"

Melanie smiles, appearing satisfied. "Nope, that's all I have."

Mrs. Morton shakes her head. "No, that's great."

"Good luck," says Dr. Armani, shaking hands with each of them.

Mr. Morton calls to the doctor as he opens the door, "Good luck on your experimental treatment. You're my only hope, you know that."

Dr. Armani turns and nods. He smiles tiredly and gives a brief wave. "Bye bye, thanks so much for coming and seeing us." Dr. Armani closes the door behind him, shaking his head. He talks rapidly to Elaine, "No prescriptions, right? Who's next?" Abruptly he shifts gears, confident that Elaine will brief Beth, who will provide the Mortons with contact information and discharge them. No tests or prescriptions need to be arranged as they do for many patients. Elaine will dictate the physician's and her assessment and plan, but she can't do it right away; sighing, she prepares to report another patient to Dr. Armani, all the while keeping an eye out for Beth so she can give her discharge instructions for the Mortons.

More than 2 hours later, as the team members finish their tasks, they leave one by one, most heading to their offices to do more work. Elaine, who is finishing dictations at a clinic desk, is the last team member in the clinic. I am exhausted, completely wasted from my day in the clinic. *How do they do this almost every day, every week?* I wonder as I leave the building.

I drive home in my sporty red car, singing along with the Indigo Girls as they harmonize on a tribute to Galileo's courage to speak the truth as he understood it in the face of damnation by the church and government.

Zooming up the interstate on-ramp, I think about forming a more structured and systematic analyses, refining the themes I have been noting in margins for months. These tentative themes and categories describe the communication I observe and participate in with the IOPOA team. I am still contemplating how the systematic analysis and my narratives will complement each other, offering multiple ways of knowing this incredible group of professionals and the remarkable people they serve. I have also been exploring my personal reactions to the team members and patients. Memories of my own illness, and my ongoing struggles with my knee pain and instability, frequently surface and blend with the events that I witness in the clinic; the lines between patient, health care provider, and researcher keep blurring.

I know I have to make some progress on my inductive analysis of communication processes in the clinic. I want to write in a way that will reflect the complexity of my experience with the IOPOA. I guess I should be nervous, but instead I am excited.

3

GROUNDED THEORY
ANALYSIS OF BACKSTAGE
COMMUNICATION

As reflected in the chapter 2 ethnographic narrative, IOPOA team members engage in a remarkable variety of communicative processes. This study uses ethnographic methods to examine a bona fide team to understand more fully how teamwork is enacted through communication. Bona fide groups occur naturally in organizations and are "characterized by stable yet permeable boundaries and interdependence with context" (Putnam & Stohl, 1990, p. 248). In this chapter, I focus on dynamic teamwork in the clinic backstage, those regions off limits to patients (Goffman, 1959).

In the clinic backstage, IOPOA team members perform social and disciplinary roles as they collaborate in providing new patient assessment and care. In the following constructivist grounded theory analysis (Charmaz, 2000; see Appendix B for a detailed description of methodology), I identify and explore inductively derived categories of backstage communicative processes. I then introduce the concept of *embedded teamwork* and explicate its relationship to frontstage (provider–patient) communication and to theorizing and administration of health care teams. To situate my findings, I begin with a summary of literature on collaboration and teamwork in health care settings.

HEALTH CARE TEAMS

———◆———

Health care teams have fostered and formalized collaboration among members of different disciplines, particularly in the field of geriatrics[1] (Lichtenstein, Alexander, Jinnett, & Ullman, 1997). Increased specialization contributes to the need for collaboration among experts from different specialties (Cooley, 1994; Satin, 1994). Composition, organization, and functioning of teams varies widely among institutions, specialties, and services provided.[2] Scholars of teamwork use differing terminology, but generally represent teamwork as existing along a continuum of collaboration. In a multidisciplinary context, collaboration is critical to the success of the program, but may be difficult to negotiate effectively because of differences in disciplinary socialization.

Representing one end of the collaboration continuum,[3] Jones (1997) defined multidisciplinary collaboration as "a multimethod, channel type process of communication that can be verbal, written, two-way, or multiway involving health care providers, patients, and families in planning, problem solving, and coordinating for common patient goals" (p. 11). Members of multidisciplinary teams work toward common goals but function largely independently, relying on formal channels (e.g., memoranda, meetings) to keep others informed of assessments and actions (Satin, 1994). Moving along the continuum toward interdependency, Wieland et al. (1996) defined interdisciplinary teams as working interdependently in the same setting, interacting both formally and informally to achieve a significant degree of

---

[1]Teams also exist in primary care (Hannay, 1980), developmental disability assessment (Sands, 1993), community mental health (Griffiths, 1998), long-term institutional care (Cott, 1998), rehabilitation (Cooley, 1994), oncology (Sullivan & Fisher, 1995), hospices (Berteotti & Seibold, 1994); and health care education (Edwards & Smith, 1998; Interdisciplinary Health Education Panel of the National League for Nursing, 1998; Vroman & Kovacich, 2002).

[2]Due to large geographical distances and/or scheduling conflicts, some interdisciplinary health care teams now work "virtually" via computer-mediated communication; technology presents its own challenges, but it also offers opportunities for effective collaboration and teamwork (Vroman & Kovacich, 2002).

[3]Representing an extreme not included in others' conceptions of a continuum of teamwork, Satin (1994) described two models of disciplinary relationships that are not defined as teamwork at all: unidisciplinary in which all tasks are carried out by members of different disciplines with no awareness or interest in the activities of other disciplines, and paradisciplinary in which awareness and courtesy exist between members of disciplines, but no coordination of efforts or joint planning takes place.

coordination and integration of services and assessments. Some role shifting and evolution may occur over time (Schmitt, Farrell, & Heinemann, 1988). In some cases, interdisciplinary teams evolve into transdisciplinary teams, in which "members have developed sufficient trust and mutual confidence to engage in teaching and learning across disciplinary boundaries" and comfortably sharing their "turf" as they work toward common goals (Wieland et al., 1996, p. 656). At their best, such teams are synergistic, enabling high-quality patient care and a high level of job satisfaction[4] (Pike, 1991).

Critics of team research argue that, despite correlations between use of teams and favorable outcomes, the effectiveness of team communication is often in doubt:

> most literature on health care teams subscribes to three basic assumptions: (1) that team members have a shared understanding of roles, norm and values within the team; (2) that the team functions in an egalitarian, cooperative, interdependent manner; and (3) that the combined efforts of shared, cooperative decision-making are of greater benefit to the patient than the individual effects of the disciplines on their own. (Cott, 1998, p. 851)

Research often fails to support the first two assumptions, and the third is unlikely to come true without the others in place.

Effective communication is crucial to teamwork but often lacking (Abramson & Mizrahi, 1996; Gage, 1998). In general, health care providers tend to strongly identify with their own discipline and its language, values, and practices (Furnham, Pendleton, & Manicom, 1981; Hind, Norman, Cooper, Gill, Hilton, Judd, & Jones, 2003; Kreps, 1988) and to relate best to members of their own discipline (Siegel, 1994). Negotiation of overlapping roles and tasks may be difficult because of territorial behavior; each team member must sacrifice some autonomy for the group to function (Sands, 1993). Role confusion, overlapping responsibilities, and other disciplinary factors can inhibit teamwork (Bateman et al., 2003; Berteotti & Seibold, 1994; Sands, Stafford, & McClelland, 1990). Successful negotiation of boundaries is a hallmark of well-functioning teams (Sands, 1993).

---

[4]Still further on the continuum, Satin (1994) proposed a "pandisciplinary" model, in which geriatrics (or another specialty) could be seen as a distinct, unitary discipline, rather than as a subspecialization across several traditional health care disciplines. In this model, team members do not represent distinct disciplines (e.g., medicine or social work), but include members sharing a unique geriatrics perspective without loyalty to a traditional discipline's values and practices. Tasks would be divided according to preference, ability, and workload rather than specialty, and training would be highly interdisciplinary.

Additionally, the ideology of teamwork often is not accompanied by egalitarianism. Despite recent changes in medical organizations, physicians remain firmly ensconced as team leaders and administrators, with the majority of the high-ranking physicians being (White) men and the vast majority of the lower status professions (e.g., nurses and social workers) being women (including women of color; Cowen, 1992; Wear, 1997). The power disparity, which is overtly a disciplinary one but often reflects traditional gender, race, and class hierarchies as well, can cause a great deal of resentment and impede successful collaboration (Lichtenstein et al., 1997). Perceptions of teamwork effectiveness vary significantly between prestigious, highly paid positions of physician and administrator and relatively low-ranking positions, such as nurses (Cott, 1998; Lingard, Reznick, DeVito, & Espin, 2002). Lower ranked team members often use strategies such as humor to resist or attenuate instructions coming from more powerful professionals on the team, without direct confrontation (Griffiths, 1998). The effectiveness of teams may be tempered through its privileging some members over others.

BACKSTAGE OF HEALTH CARE

Much teamwork among health care professionals takes place in the backstage of the health care system, where team members interact with each other away from patients (Goffman, 1959). Atkinson (1995) pointed out that health care researchers have focused the vast majority of research and theorizing of the medical practice on the frontstage of medical care–physician–patient interaction. The predominance of this focus has led to certain limiting tendencies in research. One is the relative lack of problematizing of discourse among health care practitioners that occurs away from patients. Second is a largely unreflected on preference for bounded communication episodes. Physician–patient interactions are generally brief; take place in a single, private location; and are easily recorded and transcribed (Atkinson, 1995). Such "manageable episodes" influence scholars to think of medical interactions as spatially and temporally bound.

Empirical work on health care teams clearly reflects this preference for bounded, convenient chunks of communication in its focus on formal meetings. For example, Opie's (2000) otherwise excellent study of health care teams in New Zealand centered on team meetings and excluded "joint work" between team members that occurred outside of meetings, positing that such work was only relevant to teamwork to the degree to which it was discussed within team meetings. Researchers' focus on meetings as the site of teamwork also reflects a privileging of formal, public (masculine) discourse over informal, more private (feminine) forms of discourse (Meyers & Brashers, 1994). Meetings have agendas, leaders, systems of turn-taking, and other norms associated with public communication, fitting "naturally" within researchers' existing schemas for teamwork. Such beliefs and preconceptions reflect a White, middle-class, male bias in communication research (Wyatt, 2002). Moreover, studies of meetings have traditionally focused on decision making as the crucial task of groups (Barge & Keyton, 1994). Topics such as cooperation, socialization, and connection have been marginalized, socially constructing current conceptualizations of how communication operates in small groups (and teams) that are "inherently gender-laden" (Meyers & Brashers, 1994).

My extensive interaction with one geriatric team suggests that backstage communication in the clinic is crucial to accomplishing teams' patient care goals. Using a bona fide group perspective, I sought to uncover ways in which team members engaged in teamwork outside of meetings, addressing the following research question: What are the communication processes among team members in the clinic backstage?

Although I have separated out individual processes to clarify this discussion, that separation is artificial; in practice, the processes overlap, and often a brief statement or interaction serves multiple functions. Like any other grounded theory analysis, this one highlights commonalities, patterns, and order, and it deemphasizes uniqueness, deviations from the norm, and disorder. In taking apart interactions for formulation and close examination of patterns, I am afforded the privilege of considering details at length and teasing out meanings and ambiguous functions of specific instances of communication to organize them in a schema. I have contextualized the backstage communicative processes within the complexity of multidisciplinary geriatric oncology care by including insights from interviews with team members as to their perceptions of the meanings and/or functions of some communication processes.

GROUNDED THEORY ANALYSIS CATEGORIES

In the following section, I explore backstage categories of communication individually for ease of discussion. The following seven inductively derived categories describe the communication involved in daily backstage communication among team members: informal impression and information sharing, checking clinic progress, relationship building, space management, training students, handling interruptions, and formal reporting (see Table 3.1). Due to space constraints, I selected an excerpt of the data to serve as an extended example. I will refer to line numbers periodically in the results.

TABLE 3.1   Backstage Communication Processes

PROCESS CATEGORY	SUBTYPES
1. Informal Impression and Information Sharing	Request for information/ clarification Request for opinion Request for reinforcement of message Offering of information Offering of impression
2. Checking Clinic Progress	Finding out which patients are in rooms Finding out who has seen whom
3. Relationship Building	Life talk Cancer center troubles talk
4. Space Management	Sharing resources (e.g., phones, computers) Physical movement in crowded space
5. Handling Interruptions	Patient care related (e.g., answering patients' calls) Personal or family issues
6. Training Students	Reporting Offering assistance, answering Qs
7. Formal Reporting	Reading charts Reporting to nurse practitioner Reporting to physician Writing clinic notes Dictating Communicating treatment plan and discharge instructions

Data Excerpt:

1. "Hey," said Susan [pharmacist], catching Ashley's [dietitian] eye. "Great dress."
2. "Hi! Thanks—I went on a shopping spree last weekend." She opened her white lab
3. coat further and tossed her long brown hair over her shoulder so Susan could get a good
4. look. "I bought two of these dresses in different flowered prints, both long but with
5. short sleeves, very comfortable," said Ashley.
6. Susan nodded, but then shook her head, her brow furrowed with concern. "Have you
7. seen Mr. Walker yet?" she asked abruptly.
8. Gesturing to Mr. Walker's paperwork on the counter before her, Ashley said, "I'm
9. just getting ready to go in now. Why?"

10. "He's got a real problem with his Coumadin [blood thinner] levels; they're all over
11. the place."
12. "Excuse me," said a technician trying to work his way down the crowded hall.
13. "Sure," replied Susan and Ashley in unison, flattening themselves against the slate
14. blue counter to make more room as he passed.
15. "Let me guess," said Ashley. "He's taking the Coumadin with food?"
16. "Yes," continued Susan. "And he is eating greens, you know, some days, and then
17. none on other days. I tried to tell him he has to keep a consistent intake of food rich in
18. [vitamin] K, but he didn't seem to go for it. He's stubborn. Could you say something?"
19. Ashley picked up her pen and made a note on her nutrition screening form. "I'll be
20. sure to stress that he needs to take the Coumadin by itself, not with food. That should
21. help make absorption more consistent, even if we can't get the K intake completely
22. under control. When did he say he was taking it?"
23. "With lunch," answered Susan. "I suggested midmorning or midafternoon as an
24. alternative. . . "
25. "All right, well, I'll make sure I repeat what you've said and push him to find a time
26. at least a couple of hours after he has eaten to take the Coumadin," said Ashley.

Informal Impression and Information Sharing

Informal impression and information sharing involved discussion of patients, patients' companions, and related topics. This process included five sub-processes: request for opinion, request for information/clarification, request for reinforcement of a message, offering of information, and offering of impressions. The line between fact and impression was somewhat slippery. Impressions used more emotion and description to accompany information and judgments, whereas information involved more precise, observable facts.

   Request for Information/Clarification   Team members requested a specific piece of information that was missing, in doubt, or a source of confusion. Thus, in the excerpt above, Line 22, the dietitian requested a piece of information—the timing of the medication—that she needed before speaking with the patient. An unfortunate prompt for this process was when team members discovered that patients and/or their companions had provided contradictory or inconsistent information; they then questioned each other to resolve disparities. For example, the pharmacist said to the dietitian about a diabetic patient, "I recommended that this man see his primary care physician in regard to testing and controlling his blood sugar. He said he didn't test it regularly." The dietitian replied, "He told me that his blood sugar was well controlled, and he tested it twice a day." Then the pharmacist asked, "Did he say he was taking insulin?" Through questioning each other about the information the patient supplied, the team members determined how best to address the problem.

Request for Opinion   Team members solicited opinions on issues such as affect, depression, and patients' relationships with companions both to obtain confirmation of their own uncertain impressions and to initiate discussions about patients whose perceived problems could be addressed by one or more team members' expertise. For example, the social worker collaborated when a patient did not screen at a clinical level of depression, but she sensed distress intuitively. By asking others, "Do you think she is depressed?", she effectively conducted her psychosocial assessment. Another way to request an opinion was to offer an opinion (discussed later) in a clearly questioning tone, inviting discussion. For example, after seeing a patient, the pharmacist said to the nurse, "This patient seemed frightened of her husband?"

Offering of information   Specific pieces of information about a patient and/or a companion were offered to other team members when team members perceived that such information would provide practical assistance to facilitate another team member's communication with a patient. In the earlier excerpt (Lines 10–11, 16–17), the pharmacist told the dietitian that a patient's blood thinner medication levels were unstable and that this was due in part to his diet—an issue the dietitian would be discussing with him. Mentioning that a patient was hard of hearing enabled the team member to be prepared to speak loudly and enunciate carefully. Also explaining patients' and companions' relationships avoided possible embarrassment. For example, a team member once explained that a male patient was accompanied by his sister because others assumed that she was his wife. In one unusual case, two friends accompanied a woman patient. One was a much younger man, for whom she used to work and with whom she now shared a house. He helped to care for her, but was not related to her, nor were they romantically involved. The man's cousin accompanied them—a woman who spent considerable time with both the patient and her friend/caregiver. Clarifying the relationships among the patient and her companion(s) enabled team members to better understand the patient's social support network. Similarly, researchers of a team of medical and educational specialists who provide early interventions to children with disabilities found that passing along pieces of day-to-day information informally helped team members to effectively accomplish their work (Hinojosa, Bedell, Buchholz et al., 2001).

Offering of Impressions   Team members offered each other positive or negative impressions, with or without facts to support their judgments. For example, opinions were offered of how patients were sweet, pleasant, sad, angry, uncooperative, or dominated by a companion. In the excerpt, the pharmacist described the patient as "stubborn" (Line 18). Offering negative impressions could perform a "steam-venting" function as much as a collaborative one. Two team members reported in interviews that they expressed frustration over an encounter as much for catharsis as for a desire to facilitate a team member's subsequent interaction. Venting is an important strategy for coping with stress in health care settings (Laine-Timmerman, 1999). On one occasion, an overbearing husband insisted on answering questions directed to the patient, his wife. The dietitian, social worker, and I expressed to each other how angry we felt at the husband's behavior. We did this to warn others of what they would encounter, but it was just as important to have our feelings validated by others and relieve some stress through articulating our anger. Expressing emotions in the backstage (away from patients) assisted team members in controlling their emotional display while in the clinic frontstage, thus preventing team members from disrupting the team's performance of calm professionalism (Goffman, 1959).

Request for Reinforcement of Message   This process involved asking a team member to repeat information already mentioned to a patient. Each team member was empowered to do interventions: The pharmacist made recommendations on the timing of drugs, and the social worker advised counseling, for example. To encourage patients to act on recommendations, team members asked each other to provide reinforcement, as in the interaction in the excerpt (Line 18) where the pharmacist asked the social worker to repeat her recommendation on the timing of the blood thinner medication. Another example was when patients had difficulty sleeping—due to chronic insomnia, anxiety, pain, or medications—the nurse practitioner or social worker recommended a sleeping aid. If they encountered resistance from patients who perceived sleeping aids as addictive and stigmatizing, the nurse practitioner asked the oncologist to reinforce to patients that sleeping pills are safe and effective when used properly. Team members reported that they believed that repetition increased likelihood that the patients would follow recommendations: "Sometimes it helps when they hear it twice," the pharmacist stated.

In summary, informal information and impression sharing helped break down barriers by fostering connections and overlap among disciplinary roles and tasks, moving closer to Opie's (1997) ideal of transdisciplinary teamwork. At the same time, this process helped facilitate the frontstage performance (comprehensive geriatric assessment) given by team members to patients and their companions by assisting team members in anticipating and resolving problems through backstage discussion away from the audience's hearing (Goffman, 1959).

Checking Clinic Progress

Checking progress involved asking team members which patients had been seen and by whom. With so many team and nonteam staff moving through the clinic, it was difficult to keep track of team members' locations. Team members accomplished such tracking through brief questioning (e.g., "Have you seen Mr. Walker yet?"; (Lines 6–7). Checking progress was not one team member's job; everyone took part. Angry patients or patient companions also prompted checking, as in the case of a patient and her husband who, after waiting over 2-1/2 hours, threatened to leave if the physician did not appear soon. The nurse practitioner checked to make sure that all of the other team members had seen the patient before placating the couple. The long process of assessment exhausted very ill patients, particularly those who had been undergoing chemotherapy and/or who were in advanced stages of disease. In such cases, team members requested that the nurse practitioner report on and have the oncologist see a particular patient before the others to hasten the fatigued patient's departure. A final motivation for checking progress was that nonphysician team members had competing time commitments and needed to attend to other responsibilities related to other departments or teams.

Checking clinic progress assisted team members in estimating and minimizing the amount of time before they could move on to other tasks. Although not complex, it was vital to keeping the clinic flowing smoothly. Team members valued efficiency not only for making their work easier, but also as a kindness to patients.

Relationship Building

Professional and collegial relationships rather than close friendships characterized the team, although team members' relationships varied significantly, including their relationships with me. Team members had time between patients to communicate about issues unrelated to patients. The nurse practitioner and oncologists typically had less free time than others because the oncologists saw established patients in between the new patients being seen by the entire team, and the nurse practitioner had a lengthier set of tasks and more formal reporting than the other team members. Relationship building also occurred outside of the clinic backstage as team members encountered each other in other cancer center locations during the course of their work and also in some social situations outside of work. Team members' nontask-related communication reflected two primary categories: life talk and cancer center troubles talk.

Life talk included discussing such outside interests as families, vacations, house buying, and clothing. Although topics of discussion varied over time and changes in team membership, some topics recurred. Team members who had children discussed their progress in school, sports, and other activities, sharing pictures too. The pharmacist led a children's choir and related humorous stories about choir rehearsal. When the social worker returned from a family emergency leave, team members offered sympathy and support. The pharmacist and dietitian's discussion of clothes is another example (Lines 1–5). Such talk reflects Goffman's (1959) concept of *familiarity*, where team members in a frontstage performance assume a level of informality with each other in the backstage that arises from their successful cooperation and may be inconsistent with the frontstage performance, in this case of health care professional.

The other primary category of relationship building was cancer center troubles talk (Tannen, 1990), which included mild to vehement complaining about scheduling, limited resources, overbooking of patients, overcrowding in the backstage area, and behavior of clinic staff. One source of annoyance that prompted troubles talk was the scheduling of new patients when one of the oncologists was assigned to conduct rounds for inpatients in the main hospital building. All cancer center physicians were required to take turns fulfilling this function, although it interfered with their clinics. The stress level on oncologists' rounding days was noticeably higher, as indicated by more rushing, less relationship-building talk, and impatient tones when handling interruptions. Mild griping, rolling one's eyes, and expressing fatigue and frustration were typical at these times. Team members repeatedly offered and received affirmation of the difficulty of their circumstances from each other, performing a verbal ritual of griping (Katriel, 1990). For example, "We're really hectic in here today," the nurse practitioner said to one of the oncologists as she hurried to gather materials to report a patient's case. "I know, it's crazy, don't worry," replied the oncologist. Both the team oncologists made an effort to thank the rest of the team for their hard work and patience on days with rushed schedules, which other team members reported appreciating. Both life talk and troubles talk fostered a sense of connection among team members (Tannen, 1990). Such talk enhanced collegial relations judging by the initiation of talk among team members.

Space Management

Team members shared limited space and resources with each other and with other health care providers whose practice was assigned to the clinic. A significant number of people (one approximately every 5 minutes) also passed through the clinic on the way to the break room, restroom, or photocopiers, and technicians were frequently paged to the clinic to attend to patients (e.g., conduct an EKG). The number of people in the small space made it virtually impossible to move around without bumping into others or moving into others' intimate space. Carts of patient charts and equipment also took up room. The noise level became problematic at times as phones rang, the photocopier and printer hummed, and multiple conversations occurred.

Space management involved extensive verbal and nonverbal negotiation. Nonverbal communication included claiming of desk or counter space with charts or other objects, use of facial expressions (e.g., welcoming smile or exasperated frown), pushing past someone, moving (or refusing to move) one's body to allow another to pass, and vacating when a person of higher status approached a space (e.g., chair) or resource (e.g., phone; nonphysicians made way for oncologists; administrative assistants vacated space for all other staff). The position of the door between the backstage area and the hallway of examination rooms (frontstage) was a hotly contested issue when certain people were in the clinic. Rather than openly discussing the issue, the door would be repeatedly opened and closed by the staff members according to their preference. It was not unusual for the door to be opened and closed four times in an hour, demonstrating how borders are disputed and negotiated (Goffman, 1959). This is particularly prevalent in service professions, where some team members prefer that the audience not be able to view the backstage, and others prefer ease of movement between the two regions. Verbal negotiation of space included asking how long someone would be using a computer, requesting a seat or space, (oncologists) ordering others to be quiet, move to another area, or reposition the door, and asking to be allowed to pass, as in the excerpt (Lines 12–14) where team members verbally consented and moved their bodies to accommodate the technician.

Training Students

Another of the team's communication processes involved training students in medicine, social work, nurse practitioner, and pharmacy. Students shadowed team members initially, and some then conducted interviews with patients. The team member who was functioning as a mentor for a given period of time (ranging from 1 day to 1 month) introduced her student to the other team members to initiate relationships. Training students took time and effort, although competent students in pharmacy, social work, dietary, and nurse practitioner also took on part of their mentor's workload, interviewing one out of every three patients in place of the mentor. Team members met with their assigned students before and after interactions with patients and helped with needed interventions. For example, when a social work student found that a patient needed a referral for community services, the student informed the social worker, who questioned the patient and her companion further and then made the arrangements. Social work, dietary, and pharmacy students reported relevant information directly to the nurse practitioner (e.g., drug interaction risk), with their disciplinary mentor observing the report and offering assistance only if necessary. The nurse practitioner students on their patients first to the nurse practitioner and then, with her approval, reported to the oncologist. Medical students shadowed oncologists, but did not perform any tasks or communicate with patients.

Team members trained students in their disciplines as they carried out tasks and socialized students into teamwork as they interacted in the backstage. In addition to reporting to the nurse practitioner (or, in the case of nurse practitioner students, to the oncologist), students engaged in informal information and impression sharing and relationship building with team members (and me) as we worked and waited in the clinic backstage. In Goffman's (1959) terms, students experienced both the frontstage perform-ance of providing comprehensive geriatric assessments and the backstage where that performance was dropped in favor of familiarity; they were treat-ed as people "in the know" and functioned as part of the team.

At the same time, students marked their outsider status by deferring to team members' higher status, as evidenced by students' respectful tones, waiting to be acknowledged rather than interrupting an interaction between team members, and actively listening to and carefully following instructions given by their mentors. For example, "I'm ready whenever you are," a nurse practitioner student said to the nurse practitioner, indicating she had pre-pared her report, and she would wait for a time that was convenient for her mentor. However, students were treated as trustworthy sources of informa-tion and opinions; team members requested information and opinions of students and took seriously information and impressions offered by stu-dents, often acting on them. For example, a student nurse practitioner offered to the dietitian information regarding a patient's hearing loss; the die-titian responded to the information by speaking loudly and slowly to the patient. Likewise, when a nurse practitioner student reported a patient's medical history to an oncologist, her report was accepted as the basis for treatment recommendations. Communicating in the backstage with mem-bers of other disciplines is valuable because students learn about differences in disciplinary socialization and terminology. Teamwork is increasingly important in health care as managed care decreases reliance on physicians and promotes the roles of other health disciplines to cut costs (Cooley, 1994). Teams are particularly effective at training health care students (Edwards & Smith, 1998). Having engaged in interdisciplinary collaboration during train-ing, students were better prepared to begin (or advance) their careers (Hammick, Barr, Freeth, Koppel, & Reeves, 2002; Turner et al., 2000).

Handling Interruptions

As in any other workplace, outside concerns intruded. Tangentially related and unrelated tasks were fairly minor interruptions of team members' work. I distinguish between interruptions and talk about outside concerns within the team, which I consider part of relationship building. Interruptions were either patient care related or personal/family concerns. Such interruptions were unavoidable; although they could delay patient care or interrupt team-work, they were handled efficiently. Patient care-related activities included calls or pages from team members' departments concerning patients who were not part of the geriatric program, but who were under their care in other capacities. Team members, except for the director and nurse practition-er, had only part of their time designated for the team. The rest of the time they worked with their home department and/or other teams. Thus, for example, while seeing geriatric patients, the social worker received calls that related to discharge planning for patients she served as a member of the psychosocial oncology department. Handling interruptions from other departments and teams overlapped with checking clinic progress; team members checked with others to see when they could finish their current tasks and attend to the other work. Another patient care-related task that interrupted the oncologists and registered nurses was answering telephone calls from community physicians consulting about established patients' care plans. Established patients also called the registered nurses frequently, who discussed symptoms and requested recommendations from the physicians to address patients' concerns (e.g., nausea).

Personal and family concerns also interrupted team members. Calls from child care providers about team members' sick children and pages by spouses exemplify family concerns. Nonurgent personal messages were left on team members' voicemail to be picked up at their convenience. Team members did not voice resentment of interruptions caused by other team members' personal issues, and I did not observe signs of tension between team members when one was handling an interruption. Both oncologists (the highest status team members) reported being sympathetic to the need for parents to balance work with their children's needs and expressed their understanding to team members. For example, once when the nurse practitioner received a page and had to leave the clinic to collect her sick baby at a day-care center, an oncologist smiled and said kindly to her, "Go! Go! It can't be helped. We'll be fine."

Formal Reporting

The final process I identified is the formal reporting of patient information. Team members accomplished such reporting both in writing and through oral communication, and it was both the first and last aspect of patient care. Written reporting involved reading patient charts and team-specific paperwork completed by patients and either writing or dictating a clinic note after the patient was seen. Oral reporting of information existed in conjunction with the informal system of information sharing.

Formal Written Reporting   As in all health care settings, record keeping was an essential component of patient care. Preparation for a patient interview involved looking through the chart; if available, the information provided by the patient on the paperwork was sent to patients before their visit. Information from the chart was added to assessment forms (e.g., the patient's weight was recorded on the malnutrition screening instrument). Team members attended to different types of information in the chart, with the nurse practitioner conducting the most thorough review to obtain medical history and determine patients' current stage of diagnosis and treatment.

In the data excerpt, the dietitian was reviewing a patient's chart to learn about his dietary habits, weight, and nutritional level when she was approached by the pharmacist (Lines 8–9). She added the information supplied by the pharmacist about blood thinner medication and vitamin K intake to her paperwork (Line 19).

Initial gathering of information had a profound effect on how team members constructed images of patients. According to Berg (1996), "the medical record plays an active, constitutive role in current medical work" (p. 501). Charts contain a complex but abbreviated accounting of a patient's history. Medical records reflect a biomedical assessment of the patient that relies on claims of objective data and systematic objective evaluation; records note little about how patients feel about their diagnosis, how they are coping, or what the illness means to them (Donnelly, 1988). The record not only represented past events (diseases and medical interventions), but actively shaped the current event by shaping the information team members had, what her or his expectations were, and even what blanks needed to be filled in (Berg, 1996). Thus, interacting with written accounts affected team members' views of patients before they met.

After seeing new patients, team members (except the oncologists and RNs) wrote or dictated a note—the second form of written formal reporting. The dietitian, social worker, and pharmacist wrote brief notes on the computer database while the nurse practitioner dictated the note for her and the oncologist's visit. This difference in recording medium was due, in part, to the large volume of information contained within the medical history, which the nurse practitioner dictated, as well as her responsibility for dictating some information gathered by other team members, such as the Body Mass Index (BMI) from the dietitian and the treatment plan developed by the oncologist. The selection and ordering of information determined the official accounts of "what happened" (Berg, 1996), as in this excerpt of a note written by a social worker:

> PT is a 78 YO WWF S/P liver biopsy. She is at [hospital] for evaluation by [team]. Not interested in support groups or counseling. She joined a support group after her husband died but did not find it useful. "I can do better by myself." She missed 3 of 30 on the mini mental status: She was unable to count backward from 100. She scored perfectly on the Geriatric Depression Scale. Pt denied any stressors at this time, seemed relatively unconcerned about possible treatment. Writer briefly discussed psychosocial services available at [hospital] and gave business card to PT . . . Pt is well groomed with carefully applied makeup. She emphatically answered GDS questions related to happiness.

The sense-making process of choosing details and arranging them directly affected team members' understanding of their just-concluded interactions with patients. Because team members composed separate accounts, the record generated from the initial visit could contain consistent, somewhat variable, or contrasting views of a patient depending on the amount and type of communication among team members regarding the patient. Such disparities were discovered when team members shared their summaries of patients in their weekly meeting, two to 3 days after the interaction with the patients. If disagreements warranted follow-up with a patient, a team member was assigned to contact the patients. Otherwise the divergent opinions were simply noted before discussion moved on to the next patient on the agenda; team members did not express a need to make the accounts consistent.

Another aspect of formal written reporting was the preparation of the treatment plan and discharge paperwork by the nurse practitioner and/or oncologist in conjunction with the registered nurse. Team members wrote out instructions, prescriptions, orders for tests, and other forms that were compiled by the nurse practitioner for delivery to the patient by the registered nurse. The treatment plan was also recorded on the nurse practitioner's dictation.

Formal Oral Reporting   Set reporting procedures determined in advance were completed routinely for each patient via structured verbal communication. The dietitian, social worker, and pharmacist reported specific pieces of information (e.g., GDS score) to the nurse practitioner after interacting with the patient before the nurse practitioner reported to the oncologist. The nurse practitioner then reported her own findings and aspects of the others' findings (at her discretion) to the oncologist, who then went with the nurse practitioner to see the patient. An example of a nurse practitioner dictating a case to an oncologist follows:Mr. Morton is a 71-year-old man diagnosed with multiple myeloma in 1992. Gradual onset of paralysis in his lower back and legs led to the diagnosis. Surgery was performed to remove a tumor in the vertebrae, which was then followed up with 15 radiation treatments. He had three courses of chemo that was discontinued after a liver reaction. Then he had a 96-hour continuous drip of another chemo drug, then radiation for tumors in the pelvis and femur. In February of this year, tumors were located in T5 and T6, and he began a series of seven doses of chemotherapy for those. He has had severe neutropenia and low red blood cells and was hospitalized for neutropenic fevers and cardiac problems. He says his oncologist told him that the chemo wasn't working and discontinued it, but then called him in a week later and said that blood tests show the tumors are responding. They're here for a second opinion. These are his CT scans.

Like most reports, this one focused on diagnostic and treatment information, but also included patients' perceptions and purpose for the visit.

At the conclusion of the visit, the nurse practitioner and/or the oncologist reported both the treatment plan and any orders for prescriptions and diagnostic tests to the registered nurse, who discussed information with patients and saw that they were discharged. This process of reporting was carried out for each patient. However, it occurred in the midst of other types of backstage communication, such as information and impression sharing. Thus, the social worker reported screening scores for a specific patient to the nurse practitioner, but also shared her impression that "[patient] doesn't want to continue treatment, but I think his family was uncomfortable with discussing hospice [palliative care] arrangements." For a high-functioning patient whose assessment was more a formality than an in-depth exploration, the dietitian reported to the nurse practitioner the BMI score along with her impression, "He's fine," accompanied by a casual tone and a dismissive wave of her hand. Thus, at times the ritual of formal reporting became a forum for informal impression and information sharing.

THEORIZING AND RESEARCHING TEAMS

Putnam and Stohl (1990) called for research to "improve the ecological validity of our findings" (p. 260) by paying attention to the meaning of bona fide group processes within their specific contexts—a task for which ethnographic methods are well suited (Dollar & Merrigan, 2002). Privileging formal communication (i.e., meetings) in past studies of teamwork has led to a lack of recognition of the crucial roles that informal communication play in teamwork. The ethnographic study reported here demonstrates that the clinic backstage, not just team meetings, must be recognized as a site of teamwork (Goffman, 1959).

The bona fide group model does not adequately account for the capacity for teams to interact informally through a system that they devise or adapt to suit their constraints, communication styles, and goals. The examples of interactions offered in this chapter represent the creativity of a particular team that developed ways to do its work and meet its goals more effectively. Collectively, these interactions demonstrate clearly that team members conducted significant teamwork in hallways, desk areas, break rooms, and other clinic spaces not designated as meetings. The orderly presentation of these communicative processes in the results section somewhat obscures the contextualization of the processes within the busy clinic, perhaps leading readers to perceive them as much more orderly and organized than they were. Indeed, in our interview, the team's first nurse practitioner called the backstage "controlled chaos," emphasizing that the chaos usually worked quite well in its organic development and constant readjustment. The interactions occurred opportunistically rather than on a schedule; emerged in response to team members' desires to improve patient care and assessment as they went about providing it, not by a preset agenda; were dyadic and triadic, rather than including the entire team; and developed within the process of accomplishing comprehensive geriatric assessments in an outpatient clinic, with all the noise, crowding, and simultaneously activities of that space. The opportunities and constraints differed every clinic day, and team members responded to each day's contingencies. A more holistic model would reflect this dynamism and multiple sites of communication in the everyday enactment of teamwork. Therefore, I propose the concept of *embedded teamwork*. Embedded teamwork acknowledges the discourse between dyads and triads of team members in which disciplinary (or professional) lines are blurred and redrawn; significant variation in teamwork practices occurs; team members' beliefs and attitudes are expressed and change over time; and contextual constraints are reproduced, resisted, and negotiated through communication.

Certainly, some of this negotiation of meaning happens in meetings in which ritualistic reporting of patients' cases occurs. However, the discourse of clinic practice as team members carry out comprehensive geriatric assessments should not be dismissed as joint work (Opie, 2000). Both stage models of teamwork developed by allied health and social services disciplines (e.g., Opie, 1997) and the bona fide group model that focuses on communication (Putnam & Stohl, 1990; see also Lammers & Krikorian, 1997) would be enhanced through incorporation of the embedded teamwork concept as a way to make explicit the contributions to teamwork of communication outside of team meetings. Please see chapter 6 for further discussion of the theoretical implications of embedded teamwork. In addition to the potential of these findings for theories of teamwork, this typology of backstage teamwork also offers crucial insights into frontstage health care delivery.

Bridging the Backstage and the Frontstage of the Clinic

Because of the interrelation of backstage and frontstage communication, the backstage can be conceptualized as a site for improving patient care. Backstage communication impacted communication with patients and companions in specific ways that may be useful to teams reflecting on backstage teamwork and/or considering fostering such communication. Like the typology of backstage communication, these processes overlap; they are separated for ease of discussion.

First, team members developed beliefs and attitudes about patients before they met them, and backstage communication contributed to this process. Information and opinions from other team members and from documentation in charts led to preconceived ideas about patients (Donnelly, 1988). Forming at least some ideas about patients is inevitable, and in many ways it had beneficial effects. For example, it was often helpful to know in advance that the patient about to be seen was angry or fatigued; the team member could then enter the room ready to deal with the patient's affect instead of having to react unprepared. Yet, advance warnings also may have caused snap judgments or discouraged team members from making up their own minds about a patient. For example, the social worker received negative information from the pharmacist about a couple before she saw them; being warned of the patient's husband's communication style may have helped her negotiate her tasks more effectively, but it also provided her with an unflattering impression that shaped her views. Team members did not always accept the impressions that were shared with them, however. In interviews, two team members explained that they sometimes used warnings from others as an inspiration to try to be empathetic with a patient. Health care providers should be conscious of how the information contained in charts and the information and impressions shared with them by team members has led them to anticipate certain behaviors. Ideally, health care providers should be both prepared to manage such behaviors and be open to the possibility of forming a different impression than the one fostered in the backstage.

Second, backstage communication often resulted in a modification of the agenda for a team member's subsequent encounter with a patient. The most significant and consistent example of shaping an agenda was the nurse practitioner's report to the oncologist. For every patient, the nurse practitioner had to make strategic decisions on which details to present, wanting to be comprehensive, but also balancing time constraints and not wanting to give the impression that she was unable to make sound judgments concerning what data were relevant to the oncologist's decisions. Because the oncologist had no prior contact with the patient, the oncologist's view of the patient, and hence her or his agenda, was strongly influenced by the nurse practitioner. Informal collaboration among team members also altered agendas. Recommendations that patients eliminate, reduce, or change dosages of vitamin and herbal supplements were messages that were reinforced frequently by multiple team members following backstage communication. Being prepared to address issues ahead of time, and being able to reinforce pieces of information or an impression, appeared to increase team member effectiveness and patients' receptiveness to messages. Health care providers should consider both formal and informal talk in the backstage as opportunities to adapt their own and each other's agendas for communicating with patients in ways that enhance case delivery.

Third, team members' backstage communication also provided practical facilitation of encounters. For example, being told that a patient was very hard of hearing encouraged team members to speak loudly and more slowly from the outset of their encounter and thus improved communication. Reading of patient records, one aspect of backstage formal reporting, also may have facilitated subsequent communication with patients. For example, the pharmacist always checked the list of over-the-counter and prescription medications before entering a patient's examination room. If the list was lengthy or included drugs that were likely to have harmful interactions, the pharmacist was prepared on entering the room to spend more time conducting a detailed review with the patient. Diabetics are a good example of patients who often required longer visits from the pharmacist; seeing insulin on a chart facilitated her preparation. Such practical and useful information should be freely shared among health care practitioners in the backstage to facilitate others' communication with patients.

In addition to the fairly direct manifestations of backstage communication on frontstage communication described earlier, other backstage communication processes had indirect, but significant, affects on frontstage communication. Backstage relationship building, or lack thereof, influenced team members' desire to collaborate. The nurse practitioner often had considerably less time available to engage in social talk in the backstage than other team members because of the breadth of her assessment of patients. She spent more time reading charts, recording information, and dictating than the others. How well the team coordinated their efforts and their ability to collaborate effectively affected all aspects of patient care at least indirectly. One example of this from the chapter 2 narrative was Ashley and Susan's discussion of Ashley's new dress. This type of chatting helped the two women be on friendly terms with each other and feel that the other was approachable. That approachability contributed to their willingness to seek each other out to request information or ask for reinforcement of a message. The nurse practitioners noted that they perceived themselves as having less down time, or time spent waiting, in which to engage in social talk than did the nurses, dietitian, pharmacist, and social worker, and that this contributed to them feeling less personally connected to other team members. This sentiment is in keeping with Tannen's (1990) finding that women perceive of talk as constitutive of relationships. Another example of backstage talk affecting the general atmosphere of teamwork is Dr. Armani's joke-telling; adding an element of humor to the serious business of patient care helped team members feel more relaxed and may have helped alleviate stress. Less stress could certainly enhance team members' ability to exhibit patience and a professional demeanor with difficult patients.

Life talk and troubles talk may seem at first to be a logical process to cut from the backstage to save time. However, team members seldom spent time talking when there were opportunities to complete their tasks. Clinic work was not something that could be dropped at quitting time; team members must stay until patients' visits and dictations or notes are completed, so they were motivated to be efficient. Life talk and troubles talk mostly took place on arrival, while waiting for a turn to use the computer or to see a patient, or in the course of carrying out another form of collaboration (e.g., requesting information, checking on clinic progress). Such talk also helped alleviate stress and may have helped team members cope with emotions that arise in the course of caring for patients (Laine-Timmerman, 1999). Life talk and trouble talk also had beneficial team-building effects, fostering feelings of connection among team members.

Space management also impacted on team members' abilities or desire to work with one another. Rushed schedules, cramped spaces, and insufficient computers could lead to a lack of patience with other staff. Most of this impatience seemed focused on non-IOPOA staff sharing the clinic space, but tensions also developed within the team at times. For example, the dietitian was annoyed by the lack of space for her to fill out paperwork, and occasionally the social worker grew frustrated waiting to use a computer to type notes on a patient. Several times two or more team members were kept waiting to see a patient because another team member had a particularly long interaction with a patient. Ms. Buchman and her companion, Mr. Paglio, whom I described in chapter 2, kept Ashley, the dietitian, for a very long time as Mr. Paglio described in detail every meal he had prepared for Ms. Buchman over the previous 2 weeks. This delayed the other team members and forced them to congregate in the crowded backstage area for a longer continuous period of time than usual, once they had finished seeing the other patients. They were not upset with Ashley per se, but they were frustrated at the delay and rushed to see Ms. Buchman as soon as Ashley exited the room without waiting to hear any of her feedback about the patient. Given the cramped space, I was surprised that more conflict did not arise. I often felt harassed by the frequent sensation of people touching me as they passed by or reached for something in front of me. I can see how the desire to be left alone could build and perhaps discourage attempts to seek others out for collaboration, affecting the collaborative environment. It certainly decreased my willingness to engage others in conversation on some days. Less collaboration has the potential to result in less attention to specific areas of patient care (e.g., fewer requests for reinforcement of a message).

Formal reporting in written notes or dictations is yet another aspect of backstage communication that impacted communication with patients indirectly but significantly. Because the process of writing notes was continuous, occurring between interactions with patients, making sense of one patient necessarily affected the team member as she or he moved to the next patient. That is, having determined what was important with one patient either reified or challenged existing beliefs about what was central to interactions with patients (and therefore worthy of recording). For example, thinking about depression while writing about one patient may have contributed to the overall promotion of antidepressants with patients. In one case, the social worker recognized that a man was depressed, although he did not score as at risk for depression on the Geriatric Depression Scale (GDS) and she was able to discuss his feelings with him. When she was writing a note about the man, she noted his low score on the GDS and reflected on the ways in which men of this patient's cohort were likely to respond to the items on the GDS differently than women. She reasoned that many men would not have admitted to feeling helpless, as one of the items on the scale asked, but might have responded differently if the question were rephrased. This realization influenced her subsequent interactions with patients at risk for depression. The notes and dictations thus existed in reflexive relationship with direct patient communication. The process of sense-making involved in generating the note may also have influenced a team member's communication with other team members who had not yet seen a particular patient. Thus, writing a note about a patient's weight loss problems may have reinforced to the dietitian the severity of the problem and prompted her to seek out the social worker to discuss the possibility of communal dining opportunities or home-delivered meals.

Finally, backstage communication also was central to the avoidance of negative stereotyping of geriatric patients based on their age—known as *ageism* (e.g., Beisecker, 1996; Haug, 1988, 1996; McCormick et al., 1996). Ageism appeared largely absent from team communication and communication with patients. Because their practice centers on older patients, patient age became a given, and team members made careful distinctions based on functionality, personality, social support, and other factors rather than simply age. In the course of communicating backstage, team members discussed aspects of patients' personalities, diagnoses, and treatments. Although team members had certainly developed some notions of the typical patient over time, they also noted unique attributes of patients and consciously sought to treat them as individuals. In the backstage, information and impressions were shared and negotiated, offering opportunities for stereotypes to be challenged as well as reinforced. For example, one patient and his wife regaled the team members and me with information about traveling the country in their RV to do genealogical research. Another patient played golf three afternoons a week, swam daily, and walked with her husband each evening. When Dr. Armani was called to deal with an emergency and was subsequently delayed, I had an extended discussion with one patient and her daughter about quilting. Such details of daily life helped to place the patients' illness within the broader context of their generally productive and satisfying lives outside the clinic. Team members also reported and discussed results of screenings in the backstage, such as those for carrying out "activities of daily living" and cognitive functioning. There was significant variation between patients on such scores, not consistently poor or negative scores that would have reinforced stereotypes of older patients. Low functioning patients were seen as atypical instead of normative; a very positive overall conceptualization of older adults was fostered.[5]

---

[5]Ageism also may have been less of a problem in the IOPOA than in other geriatric contexts because of the relative elitism of their patients. Although the cancer center is located in an ethnically diverse city with large percentages of Latino/a, African-American, Asian-American, and Euro-American residents, the clientele of the cancer center was overwhelmingly Euro-American women and men from the middle and

CONCLUSION

The exploration of backstage communication among members of a geriatric oncology team revealed the critical nature of teamwork *outside* of formal team meetings for both internal team functioning and communication with patients and companions in the frontstage of health care delivery. An embedded teamwork perspective offers important pragmatic and theoretical applications by complexifying the current conceptualizations of teamwork. The backstage of health care delivery will move into the frontstage of health communication research as it becomes increasingly apparent that much of the work of health care teams takes place both in the absence of their consumers and outside of formally designated team meetings.

Because the typology was developed on the basis of one team's work, the findings can not be generalized to all teamwork contexts. The elite context of a regional cancer center also limits generalizability; all but one of the team members and the vast majority of their patients were White and from middle or upper socioeconomic classes. More culturally diverse medical contexts would present constraints and opportunities largely absent in the team studied. In terms of providing a model or inspiration for future research, this study is limited by its cumbersome methodology. Although ethnography of embedded teamwork yielded valuable insights, it is time-consuming, involving long-term commitment to an organization. Researchers may find access to informal aspects of teamwork and backstage communication difficult to

---

upper classes. There were more female than male patients in the IOPOA, yet the difference was not as great as it is with the geriatric population in public hospitals, which reflects the much larger percentage of elderly women. Because older women are more likely to live in poverty and rely solely on Medicare for health coverage than older men (Ray, 1999), they are less likely to be patients at the cancer center where good insurance coverage is the norm. People of color, especially older women of color, are disproportionately represented among the poor, and hence are least likely to have the resources to travel to a regional cancer center, to have supplemental insurance, or to have a level of education that would help them navigate the complexities of the health care system.

Because most of the older patients at the cancer center are economically privileged, they are more likely to have the resources to dress nicely, to have attained higher levels of education than average, live in affluent communities, have the resources to travel, and have the resources to get attention for chronic medical conditions. Thus, they are more likely to challenge stereotypes of the elderly. Because most patients come from backgrounds similar to those of the team members, communication is facilitated by generally common expectations for language and interaction norms. There is always a gap between health care providers and patients (and their companions), but similarities and social privilege may have mediated the effects of ageism and the intersection of ageism with sexism and racism.

obtain (Atkinson, 1995; Opie, 2000). Moreover, informal interactions are not bounded geographically or temporally, and they do not lend themselves to tape-recording, making them difficult to follow and systematically document and requiring flexible data-gathering strategies (Atkinson, 1995).

Despite these limitations, the typology explored here points to the crucial nature of backstage communication in teamwork. Having presented the findings both narratively and analytically, I now turn to a highly personal account of my research and writing processes. Chapter 4 complements the analytical rendering of teamwork offered here by showing how this knowledge was constructed.

4

MAKING SENSE
THROUGH MY SENSES

An Embodied
Autoethnography

At a very simple level, the ethnographer has to sit or stand or lie or be *somewhere*. . . . A space has to be made, or found, or negotiated for the body-thereness of the ethnographer. (Coffey, 1999, p. 73; italics original)

"My body-thereness is definitely *here!*" I shout to author Amanda Coffey, tossing her book, *The Ethnographic Self*, on the floor. I have *had* it with my body. I am sick to *death* of laying around my little house recovering from my knee replacement surgery and trying to write with my laptop balanced precariously on my uneven lap. With my right leg in a huge, heavy, blue immobilizer elevated on three pillows, it is difficult to position the laptop comfortably. Actually, it is difficult to position any part of my body comfortably.

Overwhelmed by frustration and the enormity of drafting my manuscript when I cannot even make it to the bathroom without major feats of willpower, balance, and coordination, I close my eyes and let a few tears seep out. I have been rereading sections of Coffey looking in vain for inspiration that would allow me to escape this stupid body of mine and write. I just cannot seem to write anything. Day after day, I sit.

I stare at the blank screen.

I give up and read or zone out in front of the TV.

Sighing, I decide to check my e-mail account, which thankfully is accessible from my position on the couch via the wireless computer network my Macintosh-addicted husband *just had to have*. As I double-click on the e-mail icon, I have a new-found gratitude for his love of high-tech gizmos and gadgets.

An e-mail from my friend, Leigh, who shared my advisor in graduate school, waits in my inbox. I smile. I have missed Leigh very much since she moved out to Seattle to be with her partner, Jonathon. I read happily through her description of her work and what she and Jonathon did last weekend, and then I come to a paragraph that says,

> There is an article you MUST read in the new issue of The New Yorker. I can send it to you if you don't get it. It is by Stephen King and it tells about how he began writing again after a car accident. It is in the June 19 & 26 issue.

Now that is intriguing. I have sensed for awhile that at least some of my difficulty in writing chapter 4—the autoethnographic, embodied account of the clinic—stems from my current (re)immersion in the world of pain, vomit, and dependence. Being a patient is difficult for me, and to write so personally about my understanding of the clinic seems impossible from the primarily prone, pain-filled position I grudgingly inhabit these days. Somehow I can engage in systematic and detached writing, but the combination of my physical pain and the psychic wounds that accompany it are so fresh, so immediate, that attempting to dig into my body memories for insights is like rubbing salt into open wounds. Unwelcome memories of the repeated violations of my body (although done in my best interests) surface every time a wave of nausea hits or the pain spikes. I have no energy for embodiment right now.

I call my husband and ask him to pick me up a copy of *The New Yorker* at the newsstand near his office; he cheerfully agrees. As I hang up my black cordless phone, a memory surfaces. Sighing, I struggle up on my crutches, inhale sharply at the pain that this causes, and cross the living room to my bookcase. I search for the mottled purple cover of Ruth Behar's (1996) book, *The Vulnerable Observer*. Picking it up, I balance by leaning over and resting the crutches in my armpits, which is awkward but leaves my hands free to flip through the book. On page 104, I find what I am looking for—"The Girl in the Cast," an account of the year Behar spent in a cast from her mid-abdomen to her toes following a car accident, which I recalled from reading the book a year and a half ago. I hobble back to the couch holding the book between two fingers and the handle of the crutch between two others. After I rearrange my pillows and decide against the idea of struggling all the way to the kitchen for a drink, I begin reading. The alienation Behar felt from her body resonates deep within me. I read,

> But when I was told that is was time to walk again with both feet planted on the ground, I simply refused to believe that my right leg could sustain me. It didn't feel like my leg; it hung there limp, thick as molasses, unbending and foreign. How was I supposed to tell it to walk? No, it would never work. Never! (p. 112)

And later:

> The body doesn't forget. I learned to walk again, but that old fear never quite went away. It was years before I could run. It was years before I took possession of my legs. (p. 114)

Still later in the chapter, Behar mentions Oliver Sacks' account of recovering from a solitary hiking accident in which his leg was severely damaged, *A Leg to Stand On.* I immediately set my browser to www.amazon.com and ordered the book. Two days later, Sacks' book arrives via express mail, and I pry it from the thick cardboard covering in which it was shipped. Back on the couch again, I begin reading, the tension in my body ebbing slightly with each page. Yes, a small part of me cries out. "Yes," I guess I say aloud.

"What?" asks Glenn, sitting beside me on the couch, carefully studying his fantasy baseball league statistics on the screen of his laptop computer.

"Nothing, sweetie," I say absently, patting him on the arm. I keep reading. Sacks' sense of who he was in relation to his body was fundamentally altered. *It's not just me.* "I, the captain, was no longer captain," mourned Sacks, confronting his inability to control the "ship" that was his body.

Later that day, I open my copy of *The New Yorker* and read hungrily for more understanding. King does not disappoint me.

> I didn't want to go back to work. I was in a lot of pain, unable to bend my right knee. I couldn't imagine sitting behind a desk for long, even in a wheelchair . . . sitting was torture after forty minutes or so, impossible after an hour and a quarter. How was I supposed to write when the most pressing thing in my world was how long until the next dose of Percocet? Yet, at the same time, I felt that I was all out of choices. I had been in terrible situations before, and writing had helped me get over them. . . . For me, there have been times when the act of writing has been an act of faith, a spit in the eye. of despair. Writing is not life, but I think that sometimes it can be a way back to life. (King, 2000, pp. 85–86)

Well, I reason, if I am going to get back to my life, I must find my embodied voice again. I must reclaim my body and my ability to speak from it. Ah ha! *Nancy Mairs!* I struggle back to the bookcase for my copy of the antholo-gy, *Writing on the Body*, where her essay "Carnal Acts" awaits. Excited, I flip through her essay on writing as a woman living with MS, rereading sections underlined in purple pen. Then I get to my favorite part. Sighing again, but this time with happiness, I read,

> Forced by the exigencies of physical disease to embrace myself in the flesh, I couldn't write bodiless prose. The voice is the creature of the body that produces it. I speak as a crippled woman. At the same time, in the utterance I redeem both "cripple" and "woman" from the shameful silences by which I have often felt surrounded, contained, set apart; I give myself permission to live openly among others, to reach out for them, stroke them with fingers and sighs. No body, no voice; no voice, no body. That's what I know in my bones. (Mairs, 1997, p. 305)

All this time I have been trying to escape my pain-filled body to write about the IOPOA team and the patients, when what I really needed to do was allow my anguished body to speak—to claim my body and its truths.

I experienced the world of the IOPOA through my body, not just my mind, each of my senses taking it in, making sense from the sensations. I let my mind wander back over the last 2-1/2 years that I have spent with the IOPOA team.

SIGHT

> It is often difficult to know what to physically *do* in the field in order to look natural, comfortable, engaged and welcoming, while not appearing bored, threatening, or judgmental. . . . The fieldworker is a visible as well as a watching body. (Coffey, 1999, p. 73)

I shift nervously from foot to foot, not knowing what to do with myself. A smile plastered on my face, I try to look casual, as if I belong in this geri-atric oncology clinic in which I am neither patient nor staff. Having overcom-pensated for my tendency to get lost, I have arrived early for my first day of observation, and Sandra, the nurse practitioner who is my primary contact, has not arrived yet. No one seems concerned about my presence, but no one seems interested in chatting either, so I decide to jot mental notes on the set-ting—beige and blue decor, high counters and a doorway separating the staff area from the examination room area, two computers. Having assigned myself a concrete task, my nervousness recedes with each carefully noted detail. I see lots of cabinets, carts full of patient charts parked haphazardly around the desks, people in white coats walking rapidly past me down the hall, cool beige on all the walls. I pause to examine a wall with translucent brown plastic paper holders hung in several neat rows. Each holder is labeled with the type of form it contains. On closer examination of the labels, my eyes widen with recognition. Cysplatin, Leucevorin, Adriamycin—these are chemotherapy drugs.

I experience a moment of panic. Sweat beads at my hairline, and I can feel myself grow pale. *I can't do this!* I had not forgotten that I was a cancer survivor when I sought out this research opportunity, but somehow I had not thought to prepare for the emotions that were likely to surface when I entered the clinic. I try to breathe deeply, but it does not help much. Swabbing my brow with a tissue I have pulled from my purse, I concentrate on forcing my tense facial muscles to relax. A brief look around assures me that no one is watching me. I sit down on a high stool and attempt to construct a casual expression.

Sandra appears a moment later, and I stand quickly, smoothing my skirt with sweaty hands. "Good morning, Laura!" says Sandra sweetly. "I see you found us all right."

"Good morning," I say, desperately hoping I do not look as nervous as I feel. My smile feels frozen on my face. "Uh, nice to see you. Thanks for having me here today."

"Well, we are glad to have you," says Sandra. "The big guy loves to have students around," she adds, referring to Dr. Armani, the program director. I take a mental note of Sandra's tall, incredibly slim body, which is perfectly complemented by her beautiful navy dress. Form fitting without being tight, the dress gives her an elegantly professional look. She throws a white lab coat with "Sandra Bates, ARNP" embroidered in green over the pocket over it, and she sits down on the same high stool I had just jumped off. I feel frumpy in my sage green cotton knit dress, which skims lightly over my extra pounds. Through my sheer off-white stockings, the outline of the purple scars and skin graft on my right leg glow in the fluorescent light, and I wish I had worn a longer skirt.

Trying not to worry about my appearance, I lean over Sandra's shoulder as she explains to me the notes she is taking on the nurse practitioner paperwork—a set of preprinted forms designed to cover medical history, present illness, family medical history, and so on. I look up and see a woman of color, the first one I have seen so far. She is wearing a blue smock and white cotton pants. Her name tag says "Sheri Clarke, Certified Nursing Assistant." As she marks notes on a clipboard, she smiles at me, her white teeth sparkling against the background of her dark skin. I smile back, suddenly conscious of my White skin, dressier clothes, and position behind the desk. I think of the sea of White faces I had met at the IOPOA team meeting I attended last week, and it occurs to me that my Whiteness is part of my researcher tool kit—what Peggy McIntosh calls the "invisible backpack" of White privilege. How would I feel if the only other people who looked like me were the lowest paid, least prestigious workers? Would the team have accepted me so quickly if I was African American or Latina? I try again to turn my attention to what Sandra is saying about pathology reports.

Dr. Armani walks through the door, his white coat partially covering a colorful tie that features "Loony Tunes" cartoon characters. He is tall, with a broad Italian face and short dark hair sprinkled with gray. He moves quickly through the door; soon I will learn that he always moves, talks, dictates, and does everything else quickly as well.

"Hello, Laura. So good to see you today," booms Dr. Armani. He shakes my hand, and I grasp his hand firmly.

"Hi, Dr. Armani," I say, once again trying to look more comfortable than I feel. I smile brightly. "Thanks for having me."

Dr. Armani nods and then turns and scans the area. "Where is Beth?" he asks to the room in general.

Without looking up, Sandra says, "She was just here a moment ago."

Susan shrugs when he makes eye contact with her. "I have no idea," she says, returning to her own stack of papers. There is paper everywhere in the clinic—in folders, on clipboards, and stacked in piles—and a printer in the hallway churns out more almost constantly.

"OK," says Sandra, snapping her folder shut. "Let's go see Mr., uh, Frank . . . hemmer. Frackenheimer?" she says, looking at me. "I'm not sure how to pronounce his name."

"OK," I respond, happy that she has included me so I do not have to ask if I can come along. I am not versed in the etiquette of shadowing, and I hesitate to do anything that would appear intrusive or annoying. I enter the hallway of rooms, which are numbered one through six. Outside each door is a brown translucent plastic file holder, but none of them contains anything. A tall hospital scale stands against the wall near the end of the short hallway. There is also a collapsed wheelchair resting against one of the beige walls. Sandra knocks on the light wood door and then opens it. I smooth my layered brown hair and hope I look all right.

"Good morning," she calls out brightly as she enters the room. "I'm Sandra Bates, the nurse practitioner with Dr. Armani. You'll be seeing him a little later on after you see the rest of the team." Sandra shakes hands with Mr. Frackenheimer and with the woman sitting next to him. Mr. Frackenheimer is thin and wrinkled, with brown age spots peppering his pale skin. Thin gray hair covers his head and spills out of the collar of his white and beige striped golf shirt. He also wears beige pants and beige loafers and looks ready to hit the golf course, a far cry from the weak and sickly patient I had been expecting given the amount of treatment he had undergone recently for colon cancer. His brown eyes are understandably anxious, but alert and welcoming.

"I'm Mary," says the woman, offering no other explanation. I assume she is his wife. Her apricot hued hair is carefully styled, and she wears a beautiful raw silk pant suit. On her fingers are several large gold and diamond rings.

"Nice to meet you," Sandra says to her. "And this is Laura from the Communication Department who is shadowing me today. Would it be all right if she listened in as we talk?"

"Well, sure," answers Mr. Frackenheimer, nodding.

"Thanks," I say, smiling. I lean against the counter opposite Mary and listen. The counter is empty, but the cabinets above and the drawers below are labeled with the names of an assortment of medical supplies. At the opposite end of the narrow room from the door is an examination table. A blood pressure cuff hangs on the wall above it. I find myself nodding and smiling as Mr. Frackenheimer talks, although he is not speaking to me. I want to appear nonthreatening and supportive.

Sandra begins her litany of medical questions, which over time will become familiar to me. As she covers his past medical history, she asks if he has any pain or swelling in his legs.

"Well, yes I do, occasionally," answers Mr. Frackenheimer. "But it's from an old injury. I got shrapnel in my leg in the war, but it's an old pain. Twice as old as you girls!" he adds with a smile, nodding toward Sandra and me.

We laugh, and Sandra continues her questions. "How about your bowels? Are you having any constipation or diarrhea?"

"Uh, well, I was having some trouble, you know, *going*," he says uncomfortably. "So I'm, well, I'm taking some stool softeners now, and that helps. There is, the stools, they sometimes have blood in them. They are black, I mean." He shakes his head. "It's a hell of thing to talk about." Mr. Frackenheimer squirms in his seat and looks tentatively at Sandra.

"I'm glad they are helping. Lots of people use stool softeners," says Sandra casually. "We'll ask the doctor about the blood," she adds in a soothing tone. I admire how the discussion of bodily fluids, so awkward and upsetting to many patients, comes so easily to Sandra, for whom it is completely routine and a source of valuable information, not embarrassment. Mr. Frackenheimer relaxes a bit as Sandra smoothly finishes off her list of questions in casual tone, getting the details of Mr. Frackenheimer's abdominal pain and bloody stools without the slightest evidence of embarrassment or unease reflected in her face or posture.

"Do you clean your own house and cook your own meals?" asks Sandra.

"Well, actually, Mary comes over and helps me out a lot," responds Mr. Frackenheimer.

Seeing Sandra's and my looks of confusion, Mary jumps in to the conversation. "See, I'm his ex-wife. We were both married before and then widowed. We went together for 2 years and got married, but our families didn't like it at all. It was, well, it was difficult. So we got divorced, but I live right down the street, and we spend a lot of time together. We take care of each other."

I nod, and Sandra says, "I'm glad you have each other. That's wonderful." Sandra does not appear to be at all surprised by the unusual relationship. The interview concludes smoothly, and we depart, promising to return shortly with the oncologist.

Back in the desk area, I jot some notes in a pocket-sized notebook while Sandra reads another patient file. I watch Ellen, the team dietitian, move her petite frame through the doorway. She is wearing an attractive red suit that contrasts nicely with her brown curls. She is heading toward Mr. Frackenheimer's room, but I am afraid to ask if I may accompany her. Standing still, feeling awkward and unsure of myself, I continue to watch Sandra sort through a patient chart.

Fifteen minutes later, Susan catches my eye and smiles. I smile back. From the two team meetings I have attended, I know that she is the pharmacist. Mustering my courage, I turn to ask Susan if I can go with her to see her next patient. She is reading over the patient's chart, a look of concentration on her face. Chickening out, I turn back to Sandra as Dr. Armani approaches her. "Ready for Mr. Frackenheimer?" she asks him. At his nod, Sandra begins reading off of the paperwork she has carefully completed.

After about a minute, Dr. Armani waves his hand impatiently, signaling for Sandra to hurry up and finish her summary of Mr. Frackenheimer's medical history. Sandra also reports that Susan found no indication of polypharmacy, and Ellen had said that his diet was fine. "Yes, yes," Dr. Armani says irritably. "Chemo?"

Sandra consults her paperwork. "He's had four courses of Gemcidaben," she says calmly.

"Four? OK. Anything else?" Dr. Armani begins to back away, moving toward the hall of examination rooms, looking increasingly hurried and harassed.

"Well, his ex-wife is with him, and she's lovely; she helps to take care of him, and—" Sandra smiles playfully, a glint in her eyes.

"I don't need to hear about any more *lovely* companions!" booms Dr. Armani. Scared of Dr. Armani's angry look, I look around the room nervously. No one else is paying him the slightest bit of attention. I watch for Sandra's reaction. To my complete surprise, she is stifling a laugh. Looking back at Dr. Armani, I see that he is smirking. "Come on," he says, putting his arm around Sandra's shoulders and steering her toward Mr. Frackenheimer's room. It will be many months before I get used to their mode of teasing each other.

Dr. Armani enters the room first. "Mr. Frackenheimer? So nice to meet you! I am Dr. Armani!" he says cheerfully. Sandra and I follow him in and move to the back of the room as he shakes hands with Mr. Frackenheimer and Mary.

"Nice to meet you, too," says Mr. Frackenheimer politely.

"I hope you can understand me OK," says Dr. Armani. "I have been in this country 23 years, and I still have a strong Italian accent."

"Oh, I understand you just fine," says Mr. Frackenheimer, nodding emphatically.

"OK, good. Just tell me if you don't understand something. So, Mr. Frackenheimer, Sandra tells me that you have some swelling in your lymph glands."

Nodding, Mr. Frackenheimer says, "Yes, I'm afraid so."

"Under your arms, yes?"

"Yes, and in my groin as well," responds Mr. Frackenheimer.

"I see. Would you mind if I had a look at them?" asks Dr. Armani. Mr. Frackenheimer shakes his head. "Good, could you sit up here on the examination table please?"

"Sure thing," says Mr. Frackenheimer, moving up onto the table. Dr. Armani gently presses his fingers into Mr. Frackenheimer's collar bone area, then under each arm.

"OK, thank you. I need to see the ones in your groin too, please," says Dr. Armani matter of factly.

I try to catch Sandra's eye to ask her if I should leave. Before I can, Mr. Frackenheimer casually stands up and drops his pants and underwear, revealing pasty-white legs and black socks. He reveals a whole lot more than that too, but I stare resolutely at the floor, as embarrassed as if it were my grandfather standing there. Frantically, I debate whether it is better to look at him calmly as if it is common for me to see patients undressed or not to look at all. If I do not look, will that make him more comfortable, or perhaps make him feel even more uncomfortable given my thoroughly visible discomfort? I am still debating this when Dr. Armani finishes his exam and Mr. Frackenheimer fastens his pants. I have not looked, but I feel the scarlet heat on my face, and I am reluctant to make eye contact with anyone now. The rest of the discussion finishes in a blur.

As I follow Dr. Armani and Sandra back down the hall to the desk area, shame and a feeling that I blew it keep my face red and my eyes bleary. I hope desperately that I can gather my things and escape without having to talk with anyone. As Sandra and Dr. Armani discuss the next patient, I grab my purse and call out "I've got to run—goodbye! See you on Thursday!" to the room in general, and hurry down the hall, my haste making my limp more pronounced.

As I cross the wide lobby that is flooded with sunlight from a two-story wall of windows, I try to sort in my head all that I have seen, but the details remain jumbled and overwhelming. Passing an older couple on their way to the registration desk, I catch a whiff of the woman's perfume, which smells faintly of roses.

SMELL

———◆———

> Nothing is more memorable than a smell. . . . Smells detonate softly in
> our memory like poignant land mines, hidden under the weedy mass of
> many years and experiences. Hit a tripwire of smell, and memories
> explode all at once. (Ackerman, 1990, p. 5)

The pungent smell of decay hits me as I walk into the examination room, and
I struggle to keep the smile on my lips and all traces of repugnance masked.
A dark, oily stain on Mr. Holmes' golf shirt hints at a leak of some sort, a feeding tube probably, that is the source of the odor. It smells like a combination
of excrement and something that rotted in the back of the refrigerator. In the
small examination room, little air circulates, and the stench is overpowering.
I fight the impulse to cover my nose and look to Carlena for cues.

"Good morning, Mr. Holmes. I'm Carlena, the social worker who works
with Dr. Armani," says Carlena, her face giving no indication that she detects
an odor.

Mr. Holmes' face looks so tired—his brown eyes are glassy, his lips dry
and cracked. The stoop in his shoulders gives him an aura of exhaustion and
hints at resignation. "Good morning," he says softly, shaking her offered
hand.

His daughter sits next to him, and she introduces herself to Carlena. "Hi,
I'm Joyce, his daughter."

Carlena shakes her hand too. "Nice to meet you too."

I do my usual introduction and ask permission to observe, which Mr.
Holmes grants apathetically. He seems past caring about much of anything.

I look at Carlena, wondering how she will handle this. Will she question
him about the care of his tube? Will she offer help? The smell upsets me, and
not just because it is unpleasant. It disturbs me because it signals a lack of
control, an undisciplined body that cannot, *will not,* behave.

I know that feeling; it hits home with a sickening thud. I want to shout at
Carlena that she does not understand, although she is being sympathetic and
kind to this patient as she begins to work through her huge standardized list
of assorted psychosocial issues and disorders to check out. I want to say, *you
don't know how it feels to be out of control, with no hope for control, your body
taking over and not letting you be in charge. Almost past caring, you cannot quite
surrender to it.* Unwanted thoughts and memories force their way into consciousness, and I struggle to remain composed. I can feel the humiliation as
if it were yesterday, instead of 10 years ago.

I remember that I woke slowly, reluctantly emerging from the deep haze
imposed by the antinausea drugs the nurses give me during each 48-hour
chemotherapy treatment. I blinked in the semidarkness of my hospital room,

rubbing my sticky eyes and wrinkling my nose at the omnipresent smell of disinfectant. A sharp pain in my lower abdomen startled me into wakefulness, and I groaned in recognition. I searched the bed for my nurse-call button and pushed it. Glancing over at the rapidly dripping IV line, I cursed the need for continuous hydration to save my kidneys from the onslaught of toxic chemicals that was injected in that morning. The bone cancer had left my right leg a mess of grafts, stitches, and staples; there was no way I could get out of the bed, find my crutches, and hobble to the bathroom without losing control of my bladder. I was beyond exhaustion, and by the time I woke up, my bladder was so full it hurt. I would have to wait for my nurse, Chris, to bring a bed pan.

10 seconds. Please Chris, please hurry. I must remain absolutely still from the waist down or I'd lose it. I breathed fast and shallow, willing my body to obey.

20 seconds. I tightened my pelvic and vaginal muscles with every ounce of energy I could muster. *Hurry Chris, I can't hold on much longer.* This was not the first time this had happened. I recalled the humiliation of wetting my bed on two previous nights, and I fiercely vowed not to fail again.

30 seconds. My legs began to shake and tears welled in my eyes. I was losing control. It was not fair. Month after month, I endured the vomiting, the mouth sores, and the diarrhea. Operation after operation, painful procedures, and humiliating exams of every orifice filled my days. Every time I thought I could not take anymore, something else went wrong. *No*, I screamed silently, unable to accept defeat. *No!*

40 seconds. The hot yellow liquid streamed from my urethra without my consent and the searing flames of shame swept over my face. Defeated, I let the tears flow with the urine. My pelvic muscles relaxed gratefully even as my buttocks cringed in retreat from the growing wetness that surrounded them. The acrid smell reached my nostrils, and I bit my lip to keep from screaming in shame and frustration.

Chris walked in moments later and asked cheerfully, "What can I get for you, honey?" Seeing my stricken face, she immediately walked over and took my hand. "What's wrong?"

"I-I wet the bed," I said, hanging my bald head to avoid meeting her eyes.

"Oh," Chris said casually. "No problem. Let's get you cleaned up." Chris disappeared into my bathroom and returned with a damp wash cloth. "Can you sit in the chair here and wash yourself while I change the bed?" I nodded gratefully, and she helped me out of bed, wrapping her arms around my shoulders comfortingly and easing me down onto the cool blue vinyl of the recliner.

Five minutes later, Chris had stripped, sponged, and remade my bed with crisp white sheets that smelled slightly soapy. She helped me into bed and covered me up with a light blanket. I squeezed her hand in thanks and she smiled. I had been fortunate enough to be assigned to the same ward on almost every hospital admission, and I had become fond of the group of nurses who had taken care of me over the last 8 months.

"You know what?" asked Chris as she headed for the door. "I have an idea." She walked down the hall, and I stared at the ceiling with dazed eyes, pain and frustration gradually melting into tired resignation.

Chris returned with a clean bed pan, which she placed by my left hip. Raising the guard rail of my bed to keep the pan from falling off onto the floor, she said, "Now when you wake up again, you just slide yourself onto the pan, and then call me to come get it. See?"

Such a simple solution. "Thank you so much, Chris," I said, crying again, this time with relief and gratitude.

"Hey, none of that," she said with mock severity. "I'm supposed to make you *stop* crying—you want to get me in trouble?" Chris slipped out of the room as I smiled through my tears.

I smile at this memory, despite the pain, able to see the hope and comfort as well as the hurt and powerlessness. Returning my attention to Mr. Holmes, I cannot shake the overwhelming desire to *fix* the problem—to get his body back under control. My heart breaks for him, and at the same time I want to tell him not to give up. It occurs to me that it is for *my* sake that I wish him not to give up, not for his—to make it easier for me. Ashamed of my thoughts, I look down at my feet. The smell still bothers me, but I am able to ignore it for the most part as Carlena continues her questioning and screening for depression and cognitive functioning deficits. Later in the visit, Sandra will question Mr. Holmes and his daughter about the maintenance of his feeding tube, offer advice on caring for it, and suggest that he see his primary care physician as soon as possible to have the tube thoroughly checked.

When I return home that afternoon, I feel a complex mix of shame, sadness, anger, and helplessness. I think of Arthur Frank's words and reach for his book, *The Wounded Storyteller*. Taking it to a comfortable chair, I scan until I find the section I am looking for.

> Illness is about learning to live with lost control. . . . When adult bodies lose control, they are expected to attempt to regain it if possible, and if not then at least to conceal the loss as effectively as possible. . . . The work of the stigmatized person is not only to avoid embarrassing himself by being out of control in situations where control is expected. The person must also avoid embarrassing others, who should be protected from the specter of lost body control. (Frank, 1995, pp. 30–31)

"The specter of lost body control," I repeat aloud to myself. The term *specter* connotes a visual image—spectacle. Yet loss of body control can also manifest as auditory and, most definitely, olfactory. Indeed, smell is a much more troublesome indicator of loss of control than appearance. A spectator can shut her eyes or look away, but she must continue to breathe. The scent enters the body of the others who perceive it, carried by water vapor into the nasal cavities, threatening the witness in a far more personal, more immediate, manner than a sight could. Like a loss of control that is tactile, which involves touching another inappropriately, smell confronts the other where she or he lives—*in a body*. As I mull over the strong odor of the patient, it occurs to me that smells are difficult to put into words.

A week later, I am back for another day in the clinic. I am exhausted just thinking about spending the next 4 hours standing on my aching knee. Today's clinic begins at 11 a.m. rather than 9 a.m. because Dr. Armani is doing hematology rounds in the main hospital building this week. As always, I arrive in the examination room hall through the door that connects to the lobby and proceed down the hall to the desk area to stow my purse. Breathing deeply, I notice how cold and dry the air-conditioned air is in the clinic. The windows in the lobby let in so much light and heat that the thermostat compensates by running the air conditioner at full blast all day long. This results in a comfortable temperature in the lobby and a very chilly one for the clinic examination rooms and staff areas. Several times I have fetched blankets and draped them over the shoulders of chilled patients as the air conditioning brought the temperature in the examination rooms seemingly to Arctic levels.

"Hi!" calls Susan as I enter the desk area. I look down the hall to my right and see her using the photocopier.

"Good morning," I say, walking toward her. "What's up?"

"Not much, just making some copies," says Susan cheerfully. "How are you?"

"Pretty well, thanks," I reply. "A little tired."

"School wearing you out?" asks Susan sympathetically.

"Yeah," I say, not adding that while teaching and writing papers are tiring, they pale in comparison to spending even a few hours in the IOPOA clinic. The sharp odor of hot toner wafts up from the copier as Susan continues copying documents, and it does nothing to enhance my dreary mood. I try to psyche myself up for the next several hours of observation, telling myself how interesting the team and patients will be today, but all I can think of is how tired I am, physically and emotionally, and how much I would rather be at home on the couch watching television with a big mug of chai tea.

Although observation is interesting, and I feel like I am learning a lot, I am having more and more difficulty handling the helplessness that almost overwhelms me as I continue to meet patients and their loved ones. My inability to aid these people evokes painful feelings of powerlessness and grief from my own early days of diagnosis and treatment decision making. I cannot take away their pain anymore than I could take away my own or my family's. Over and over I write in my notes, "I feel helpless," "I wish I could do something to help these kind and brave people," "I am completely powerless." The lack of control exhausts me. Forcing my attention back to the conversation, I nod as Susan tells me about how busy and understaffed they are in the infusion center pharmacy where all the chemotherapy dosages are prepared. Susan misses or is late to IOPOA team meetings fairly often because she cannot get away from the pharmacy.

"I keep telling my boss I need coverage so I can keep up with my team responsibilities, but they're never going to allot the money to hire more staff," says Susan, clearly frustrated. "The system here stinks."

Knowing how seriously Susan takes her responsibilities, I am sympathetic. "I know they keep you awfully busy. It must be hard for you to have to divide your time among the IOPOA and the infusion center," I say with genuine concern.

"Well, it is. The IOPOA stuff is supposed to take priority, but what am I supposed to do when there is no one to cover me?" Susan shrugs off her frustration good-naturedly, or perhaps resignedly, as she organizes her folders and documents. "Better get cracking. Do you want to come with me to see Mr. Tash?"

"Yes, that would be great. Thanks," I say, stepping back to allow Susan to precede me. We pass Ellen on the way to Mr. Tash's examination room. She is bent over a stack of dietary screening forms, eating spoonfuls of low-fat cottage cheese alternating with bites of tropical fruit-flavored applesauce. The fruity scent is far more pleasant than the toner, and I take a deep breath of it before greeting her. "Hi Ellen!" I say brightly.

She looks up at me from her seat and smiles. "Hi! How are you?" she says. Her tone is friendly but she looks distracted, and I feel kind of bad for interrupting her.

"I'm fine," I say, without stopping. "How about you?"

Already turning back to her paperwork, Ellen calls over her shoulder, "Fine, thanks. Busy."

We pass through the doorway and into the examination room hall. Susan consults her list. "He's in Room 3."

The thought of meeting yet another friendly person with a deadly disease pains me. Sighing, I have to force a smile as Susan knocks on the door. She pauses. Patients often call out "Yes" or "Come in," but this time we hear nothing. Susan opens the door part way. "Mr. Tash?" she says tentatively, perhaps concerned that another team member was already with the patient.

Mr. Tash calls out cheerfully, "Come on in!" We enter the small room, and I see Mr. Tash and a woman sitting in chairs, side by side, holding hands and grinning widely.

"I'm Susan, the team pharmacist," says Susan, extending her hand.

Shaking her hand, Mr. Tash chuckles. "Did you think we were smooching in here?"

"No, no," says Susan, laughing. "I thought another team member might be with you. Are you Mrs. Tash?" she asks, shaking the woman's hand.

"Yes, nice to meet you," says Mrs. Tash, also chuckling.

Winking conspiratorially, Mr. Tash adds, "She's a good smoocher, you know." He smiles at his wife fondly, and she pats his knee.

"Well, that's important!" says Susan, and we all laugh. As I lean forward to shake Mr. Tash's hand, I inhale his light, fresh scent—a pleasant mixture of soap and a spicy aftershave. The Tashs' faces glow with hope, love, and good cheer, and I find myself smiling with genuine cheerfulness in return, feeling more peaceful than I have in a long time.

Two weeks later, I am conducting audiorecording in Dr. Klein's clinic. I have finally succeeded in getting approved by both the hospital Scientific Review Committee and the university Institutional Review Board to tape record interactions between staff and patients. I am hoping that the transcribed interactions will complement my fieldnotes with an in-depth look at a small number of patients. Unfortunately, I have had limited success recruiting patients, which puzzles me. Since my arrival, the vast majority of patients have been eager to share their stories with me and even just to have some company during their long visit. All that changed when I whipped out my informed consent forms and tape recorder. I am mulling this over as I pull into a parking space and hustle across the lot as quickly as my aching leg will take me. A groundskeeper is mowing the grass this morning, and the sweet smell of freshly cut grass fights a losing battle with the noxious odor of the mower burning gasoline as I approach the door to the building.

I am late; *I don't know what I was thinking.* To recruit patients scheduled for 9 a.m. appointments, I need to get to them in the waiting room by 8:30 or 8:45 so as not to interfere with the operation of the clinic. For some reason, that did not compute in my brain this morning, and I was thinking I did not need to arrive until 9 a.m. It is now 8:50. As I rush through the waiting room, I can feel the sweat running down my face and dab at it ineffectually with a tissue. So much for the carefully professional persona I hoped to convey. I am wearing a light woven blouse in pale lilac and a black skirt that features flowers in the same lilac as well as sage green leaves. I enter the bathroom to wash my reddened face, and I notice a much darker shade of lilac has stained my entire back. The odor of sweat mixed with the scent of my deodorant wafts up to my nose as I try to blot my soaked back. I want to cry in frustration. I wish I could will the flush from my face and the sweat from my back. I pull myself together as well as possible and leave the sanctuary of the bathroom reluctantly.

The nursing assistant has already brought the patients back into the examination rooms, and I saw from the posted list that one of the three had canceled, so I head into Room 4 to find the next patient on my list, Mr. O'Reilly. The older man seems exhausted and I hate to bother him, but I begin my schpiel anyway. His highly anxious sister is sitting with him and frowns throughout my explanation, drawing her cardigan sweater more tightly around her in the stale, chilly air. I shiver as the air conditioning blows unceasingly into the room and the sweat on my back turns cold and clammy. He says yes despite her concerns, and then as I am struggling to hurry to get the tape recorder set up, I cannot get the tape to start and I mutter something under my breath. Suddenly, Mr. O'Reily decides this will be too much bother. "I don't want to do this," he says.

His sister immediately jumps in, "This is too intrusive. It's going to get in the way."

Close to screaming with frustration, I say as calmly as possible, "No problem, I understand. That's fine. I hope your appointment goes well." I gather up my equipment in my arms as I say this, trying to smile and sound sincere, but probably failing. I can feel the cold sweat still rolling down my back. I walk back to the desk area, cursing the oppressive summer heat and miserably wondering just how sweaty I smell. Beth is already seeing the only other patient for the morning. *Fine, just fine*, I think sarcastically. Susan approaches me and asks, "I am going to see Mr. O'Reilly—he's your patient for today, right?"

"No," I say, sighing. Dr. Klein pauses and turns toward us, listening to my explanation. "He decided he didn't want to do it. Said it was going to get in the way." I try to back up slightly, conscious of my perspiration and hoping the scent is not strong enough for them to notice. None of the team members ever appears sweaty.

"Oh, well that happens," says Susan sympathetically.

"Yeah, well," I say, shrugging impatiently.

"Are you going to try another patient?" she asks.

"There *isn't* another one," I say more sharply than I intend. Taking a deep breath of the chilly air, I continue my explanation in a more pleasant tone. "One canceled, and the other is in with Beth now." Trying to look on the bright side, I shrug and add, "Well, this gives me some time to get some other things done."

Dr. Klein smiles at me and says reassuringly, "Ah. Recruiting patients is often difficult and slow. We have this problem too with our studies." She nods encouragingly.

I smile back at her, grateful for the support, but my clammy back, my sweaty brow, and my embarrassment are too much, and I cannot keep the frustration out of my voice. I am embarrassed by my failure to recruit and by my still sweating body. "I knew it would happen this way sometimes. I just want to get this taping over with sooner rather than later."

Dr. Klein laughs softly; she is not laughing at me, but with me, inviting me to shake off my disappointment for the day and join the laughter. *You can't control everything*, she seems to be saying, *so don't worry about it*. I give it a try, grateful that the team members appear nonjudgmental of my ineffective attempts to recruit patients. As I stuff my equipment into my bag and wave goodbye, I think about control again—about wanting to force my body to do what I want it to do, about the way the medical system forces patients to surrender control of their bodies, about Mr. O'Reilly who asserted a small degree of control when he withdrew permission to record his visit, about my desire to control my study.

About learning to live with lost control.

SOUND

The sharp ring of the phone startles me as I sit reading a stack of articles on multidisciplinary health care teams, all of which are dry but contain important information I need to ferret out. I grab the black cordless phone that rests next to me on the blue and beige striped couch.

"Hello?" I say.

"Laura? This is Sandra. How are you?" says the familiar voice on the other line.

I smile at Sandra's warm tone; I have liked the IOPOA nurse practitioner since the moment I met her. "Hey Sandra. I'm fine, how are you?"

"I'm well, thanks." We chat for a bit about my classes and her baby, and then she gets to the point of her call. "Listen, I had to call to give you some news," she says with considerably less enthusiasm.

"Uh, shoot," I say warily, my mind conjuring up all sorts of horrible things, such that she is sick or that the hospital has decided not to let me continue my research.

"I just resigned my position at the cancer center," she said.

I am disappointed, but not shocked. She has been balancing so much for so long—an infant, a husband who travels extensively, pursuing a Ph.D. in anthropology, and working 50 hours a week with the IOPOA. "I'm so sorry to see you go," I offer, not sure what to say. Selfishly, I wonder, *what is this going to do to my access?*

"Thank you. I will be filling in from time to time," offers Sandra. "I already told Elaine, the new nurse practitioner, about you. I'm sure you'll be fine together."

I am not so sure, never having met her, but I don't say so. "Oh, I'm sure we will," I respond, my voice miraculously sounding much more confident than I feel. Before we hang up, we chat for several more minutes about her plans to devote herself to finishing her Ph.D. in medical anthropology and to raising her son.

Now it is my first day in the clinic with Elaine, the new nurse practitioner. I am scared that if she does not like me, she will ask me to leave. I have no reason to think she would do any such thing, as she has been very cordial to me in my contact with her at staff meetings and during a brief conversation in her office. But I am still scared. Sandra made my presence in the clinic so easy in so many ways, introducing me to patients, always offering to have me accompany her, asking if I was getting what I needed. *I don't know what I need,* I want to cry now, the focus of my study still vague after a year of observation. *And if I did, how would I go about getting it without Sandra's help?* Moreover, the social worker with the team, Carlena Newman, declined to return after maternity leave following the birth of her second child this summer, so the team has a new social worker, Joyce Fitzgerald, whom I met at the last staff meeting. Only a few months later, Ellen, the dietitian with the team, would transfer to another program, and I would have to get to know the new dietitian, Ashley, as well. Lucky for me, both of the new team members were warm and supportive of my presence, just like Elaine turned out to be.

Still, on this, my first day back in the clinic after a busy summer of teaching, taking classes, and working on a research project with Sandra, I am more than a bit nervous.

"Good morning," I say with enthusiasm as Elaine walks in the door to the staff area.

"Good morning," she says cheerfully. Elaine slaps a pile of charts on a desk and then looks up. "How are you?" Elaine's voice is pleasant, but very different from Sandra's soft southern accent. Elaine sounds very straightforward and efficient, polite but no-nonsense.

"I'm doing fine, thanks. And you?" I say, trying to sound friendly and confident.

"Oh, pretty well. It's going to be a busy day," says Elaine.

I nod and hope I sound sympathetic as I say, "Yes, I'm sure it will be." The clinic is crowded, and I feel in the way standing in her narrow passageway between the desk and the high counters, so I move to stand behind the counter. To my right, a doctor views CT scans on the light board while listening to information from his primary nurse. Dr. Armani is on the other side of him, roaring into the telephone, but I have no idea who has incurred his wrath. An administrative assistant types and clicks her way through a series of computer screens, calling up test results for one of the patients.

Susan greets me warmly as she walks in. "Hi! We haven't seen you in the clinic for awhile. It's good to see you."

"It's good to see you too," I say, hastening to explain my absence. "I have been teaching summer school and taking classes and then I went on vacation, so I haven't been available."

Susan nods, "I figured something like that. Well, glad you're here."

"Thanks, me too," I say. It has been 8 weeks since I have ventured into the clinic, and I feel very uncomfortable. I try hard to make my voice sound assured, as if I were certain I am welcome and belong here, but I only sound defensive.

All the team members and other staff working in the clinic go about their business as if I was not there. I stand close to a wall, trying not to be in the

way. I am afraid to ask Elaine or Joyce if I can accompany them, and this discomfort makes me uneasy about asking Susan or Dr. Armani either, although
I know them pretty well. I listen to the hum of the clinic as the morning
wears on. My discomfort increases as I continue to stand in my corner, trying to display comfort with myself. Not having accompanied anyone to the
first patient he or she saw, I now feel even more reluctant to ask to accompany them to their next one, afraid that they will think I am being intrusive.
Beth chats with me in between returning several patient calls, which I enjoy.
I can hear pagers going off every couple of minutes, their high-pitched tones
irritating in their persistence. I am the only person in the clinic who does not
carry one, and I am grateful to be exempt.

Thinking of the sharp sound of pagers rips open a scab I had not known
still lingered on my psyche, and I gasp as the blood/memory flows.

It was the worst night of my life.

Ten months into my chemotherapy and following a series of infections,
I had passed out while staying with two friends. Jim and Garry all but forced
me to call my doctor, who insisted that I go to the hospital for tests. I was
admitted late on a cold early December afternoon, twilight already descending on Burlington, Vermont, although it was only 4 o'clock. Almost 8 hours
later, I had been poked and prodded, stabbed and stuck, and the frantic resident in charge still had no idea what was wrong with me. I had a fever of
103 and virtually no white cells. They took blood cultures, did a spinal tap,
and examined every inch of my body. Residents, interns, medical students,
and nurses moved in and out of my room quickly, their pagers emitting their
irksome whine over and over. No one talked to me. They did not seem to talk
to one another either, as I was asked the same questions over and over. On
the few occasions when the staff addressed each other, they did it across my
bed, as though I was their anatomy class cadaver.

As I lay exhausted on my bed, staring blankly at the beige wall in front
of me, the tall, brown-haired female resident burst into my room again, two
more medical students hovering in her wake. "OK," she said decisively. "We
are going to remove your Porto-Cath.[1] Let's get you prepped for surgery."
Offering no other explanation, she yanked my blanket down off my chest
and began to listen to my heart.

Startled and offended by her abrupt manner, something inside me
broke. I had had enough. "No, you are not," I said slowly, carefully. "No one
is doing anything else to me until someone tells me what is going on. What's
wrong with me? Why would taking out my Porto-Cath help?"

---

[1]A Porto-Cath is a device that is surgically implanted beneath the skin to enable infusion and blood drawing. It is a metal disk with a hard rubber center that can be
accessed through the skin with a needle. Attached to the disk is a catheter that is
implanted into a sizable vein. Porto-Caths and similar devises are routinely provided
for cancer patients and others who have frequent infusions.

Her eyes wide in fury, the woman, who in 8 hours had not volunteered her name, screamed at me, "*Do you want to die?!!* Because that's what's going to happen if you don't let us take this out! *Is that what you want?!!*"

I cried tears of sadness and anger. "No," I managed to choke out. "No, I don't want to die. But I do want to know what's going on."

Glaring at me, the woman turned on her heel and stomped out, the nervous medical students shuffling behind her. I did not try to fight the sobs that wracked my weary body. Attracted by the yelling, my nurse, Steve, came to my door. When he saw me crying, he wordlessly put his arms around me and I sobbed into his shoulder.

When I was through, he handed me a wad of tissues and asked what happened. I told him. Patting me on the hand, Steve turned and silently left my room.

Moments later I heard his deep voice echoing in the hallway. "What the HELL are you doing, yelling at that girl? Do you have ANY idea what she's been through? DO YOU? And you think it is going to help to SCREAM at her?"

A mere hint of a smile formed on my lips as Steve's yelling continued. I felt the warmth of his caring, and although it did not make the hard night go any faster, it helped me to find the strength to make it through until dawn. That resident never apologized for her unkindness, but she did come in and give me as thorough an explanation of what was going on as she could provide. Eventually I was diagnosed with septicemia, the spreading of the infection in my leg to my bloodstream.

With memories like this one, it is no wonder that I have resisted the perspectives of the medical personnel and continued to embrace the patients' points of view. Yet I have never seen an IOPOA team member treat a patient cruelly or even unkindly. I do not think of Elaine, Dr. Armani, or any of the others as the one-dimensional monsters or angels of mercy like some of the doctors and nurses who live on in my memory. Sighing, I stuff the feelings down, reminding myself that I do not have time for such memories right now.

Scanning the room, smiling a smile I do not feel, I watch the team and other personnel go about their tasks. I do not usually spend so much time in the desk area because Sandra always introduced me to patients and got me started almost immediately in talking with them. Often I would simply stay with a patient as the team members came and went. Despite my discomfort, the almost 2 hours I have spent standing around this morning have begun to yield an inkling of an idea—a new understanding. I have been so focused on communication with patients (i.e., with the people I identify with) that I have not paid much attention to the communication in the desk area.

The phones ring incessantly. "Med Onc," says Beth as she answers the one nearest to her, using the abbreviation for "Medical Oncology Clinic." "He's in with a patient right now, can I take a message?" As she reaches for a note pad, I look over to Elaine, who is listening to a report on a patient from

Brenda, a nurse practitioner student. Joyce and Susan are talking about a patient. I lean over to listen.

"He clearly has short-term memory loss," says Joyce.

"Well, his medications are *completely* messed up. I thought he might have a memory problem. He doesn't know when to take anything." Susan shakes her head. "Someone else needs to be in charge of his medications."

Joyce nods. "I talked with his daughter about it and suggested that she get one of the those pill boxes with the different days, so she can lay out all the medications for him."

"That's a good idea," agrees Susan. "I'll talk to Ellen and see if she found whether he is having trouble cooking for himself. I know he lives alone. If his memory isn't good, he may not be eating well either."

"Yeah, that's a good idea. He told me he was eating fine, fixing simple things, but let's go talk with Ellen to be sure. She should have a better idea of what exactly he's eating." Susan and Joyce walk together over to where Ellen is giving some numbers to Elaine, who has stopped talking with the student long enough to jot the nutritional risk screening score on the patient's chart. I see the three of them talking together, and it makes me think. I get out my palmtop computer and begin typing as rapidly as the miniature keyboard will let me.

I had always viewed the backstage area as a holding pen of sorts—an area to wait in until you could see a patient and a place to document patient data. Yet now as I listened carefully, I was hearing much more. The team members talked with each other about patients, sometimes seriously, and other times in more casual conversation, often with great emotion, as they vent frustration, anger, or sadness.

As the day goes on, I become an eager eavesdropper, a wicked girl of whom my grandmother would disapprove. I cannot shake the feeling *that I am not supposed to be hearing this stuff;* I am a patient, not a team member. It suddenly occurs to me that I am hearing discussions similar to what must have gone on outside my hospital room and what continues to happen in the consultation room when I see my orthopedist. I pop open my palmtop computer and begin typing on the tiny keys, slowly at first, but with increasing speed.

It is like being allowed backstage at your favorite musical, the one that moves your very soul, even though the story is tragic. But when you get back there, you see all this stuff you aren't sure you wanted to see. You didn't want to see that all the actors have bad days and near-misses and friendships and alliances and scripts and props. You didn't want to see the back of the carefully painted scenery. On the other hand, you have an even greater appreciation for what they do on the stage, for how they pull it off, day after day, show after show. It is just so much more complex, so messy, and yet so beautiful, in some ways. You see the scaffolding, and it helps you to understand more deeply the performance that occurs on the stage. You are overcome with the guilty pleasure of viewing the forbidden zone in which the masks come off . . . or perhaps they are only traded for other masks.

"Excuse me," says a familiar female voice, startling me out of my written reflection. I jump back, making room for the woman to pass, and notice that it is Muriel, the registration specialist.

"Hi Muriel," I say with a smile.

"Oh, hi. How are you?" she asks, recognition dawning on her face.

"Fine, and you?"

"Just fine." Muriel holds up a bag and adds, "On my way to lunch." She waves and continues down the hall to the break room, the bag rustling softly as she walks. I snap my computer shut and slip it into the pocket of my crisp blue linen blazer.

I scan the backstage space. Elaine is writing down numbers that Ellen is giving to her for two of the morning's new patients. Joyce is typing a note at one of the computers, the gentle tapping of the keys barely audible amid the numerous voices and other sounds of the clinic. Beth is describing a problem with one of the established patients to Dr. Armani, seeking his recommendation so she can call the patient back.

"OK," says Dr. Armani. "Call in a prescription for Oxycontin for her."

"Twenty milligrams, twice a day?" asks Beth.

"Yes," confirms Dr. Armani. Smiling, he adds, "Beth, I have a new joke for you!" He looks around quickly to see if there are any more takers; he loves an audience. One of the other doctors obliges and ambles over to where they stand. I stay where I am, but turn my head to listen. "What do Monica Lewinsky and Hillary Clinton have in common?" asks Dr. Armani.

"What?" ask Beth and the doctor in unison.

"Hi, Laura! It's nice to see you," says Ellen from right behind me, drowning out the punch line. Beth and the doctor laugh. I turn to smile at Ellen, noticing how much larger her belly is than last time I saw her. She is now in the third trimester of her pregnancy, and her rounded abdomen is emphasized by her otherwise petite frame. I had seen her earlier from the other side of the high counter and had not noticed the dramatic change that 2 additional months of pregnancy had brought.

Thinking to myself that I will have to ask Dr. Armani to repeat the joke later, I greet Ellen. "Hi! You are looking healthy. How are you and the little one feeling?"

"Oh, good," she says, patting the sheer Rayon fabric that ensconces her belly. "Getting bigger," she adds with a chuckle.

"That's great," I say.

Susan approaches and asks Ellen about Mrs. Dobson. "Did she tell you she was taking 800 IU of vitamin E per day?" she asks, holding up the phar-

macy paperwork that Mrs. Dobson filled out before her visit. The dose of vitamin E is printed neatly in blue ink under "vitamin and herbal supplements."

Ellen nods, looking exasperated. "Yes, I told her that she should be taking no more than 400 IU since more than that can be toxic."

"What did she say?" asks Susan.

"She said she went to a nutritionist who prescribed that amount. It's supposed to enhance her immune system," says Ellen, skepticism permeating
her voice.

"Never mind the potential for toxicity," says Susan sarcastically. Shaking
her head, she continues, "I'll try to persuade her too."

Ellen replies with a shrug, "Good luck."

Leaning against the high counter in a vain attempt to ease some of the
pain in my knee, I wonder what Ms. Dobson would think of the team members strategizing about her behind the scenes. Most likely, she has no idea
such communication goes on. I know I never did as a patient, before beginning my research. Certainly, she will never have the opportunity to participate in, or even listen to, backstage team discussions of her case.

I stand there thinking, looking in vain for an empty seat, while trying to
look as if I am not needing to sit. One of the administrative assistants
approaches me. "Hi!" she says as she passes.

"Hi!" I respond, automatically smiling and moving closer to the counter
so she can get by easier. Resuming my rumination, I think back to just last
week when I went in for a checkup with my surgeon, Dr. Rose, who recently moved his practice from the clinic where I had begun seeing him over a
year ago to the Southeast Regional Cancer Center. It was eerie to register as
a patient at the institution I had been studying for over 2 years, although it
was in a different building than the one in which the IOPOA clinics are held.
Having been duly processed, assigned a number, and issued a gray plastic
hospital identification card, I walked to Dr. Rose's waiting room.

An hour later, I sit on a paper-covered examination table, my blood pressure, weight, and temperature freshly recorded on the chart that rests on a
bedside table in front of me. My husband sits in a chair next to the table,
smiling supportively. I see Dr. Rose walk into the consultation room, the main
backstage area in this clinic space. On his heels is his current fellow or resident. They shut the door, and I am more than a little curious about what they
are saying about me. Despite my deep fondness for Dr. Rose, an incredibly
kind physician who listens to me respectfully and supports me in making
decisions, I suddenly feel anew the relative powerlessness of the patient. I
know the patient role well and play it perfectly. I do not have the freedom to
move about the clinic; I sit and wait for the busy physician in the small room
I have been assigned. I sit where I am told, bend my knee when requested
to, answer questions I am asked. I need his expertise, and I must trust him
to have my best interests at heart and sufficient knowledge to help me get
better. The contrast between my performance as patient and my perform-

ance as privileged researcher is uncomfortably sharp, and it makes me uneasy. No matter how benevolent the power held by health care providers, it is magnitudes higher than that of patients.

I quickly set aside this unwelcome awareness as Dr. Rose enters my room, smiling cheerfully. I feel the warmth of his strong hand as it envelopes my smaller one in a firm handshake.

TOUCH

My knee throbs dully as I continue to stand in the desk area, leaning slightly against one of the high counters. Susan walks over and gives me a hug. I hug her back gratefully. Another tiring day, and yet she makes me feel so welcomed. Susan began hugging me periodically after my first year of observation. She is always friendly to me, even extending me an invitation to a "Pampered Chef" party she was hosting. I have been feeling increasingly at ease with team members as I spend more time with them. Joyce and Ashley invited me to go out for drinks with them and some friends after work one day. I have also spent considerable time outside the clinic with Sandra, both discussing our research projects and just socializing.

Leaning on the high counter, I keep an eye out for an empty chair. Joyce walks through the door, her face reflecting a deep sadness. When I smile at her, I get only the slightest of smiles in return. "Hi," I say. "Are you OK?" Tentatively, I touch her forearm lightly, trying to communicate my concern.

Joyce nodded. "I'm just sad. I just saw Mr. Werner. He is so sweet, and his daughter and son-in-law were with him. It just doesn't look good. He's trying to take care of his wife; she's demented and needs a lot of care." Joyce shook her head. "He has stage four chondro sarcoma, with metastases to both lungs. He probably won't live long."

I nod and murmur, "That is sad," not knowing what else to say.

Ashley, the dietitian who replaced Ellen on the team a few months ago, nods too. "How sad," she says to Joyce. A look passes between them, and Ashley places her hand lightly on Joyce's shoulder before gathering up her stack of paperwork.

I am surprised at how sad I feel, and I have not even met the man and his family yet. I am caught between a deep curiosity about this man whose disease is very similar to the one I survived and a sense of embarrassment at having not only survived but become a researcher of the context I was once so much a part of as a patient. I decide to try to meet him, especially because Joyce said he was so amiable despite his poor prognosis.

"Ashley, are you going to see Mr. Werner now?" I ask.

"Yes," Ashley says. "Would you like to come along?"

"Very much, thanks." As we walk down the hall, I add, "He has a form of cancer very similar to the one I had."

"Oh?" says Ashley, her eyebrows raised in surprise. "That must be weird for you."

"Mmmm," I say noncommittally. "Kind of." I don't say that it is also kind of exciting and scary and guilt-inducing at the same time. I think of Arthur Frank's term, *the community of pain*—those who are connected by a shared knowledge and experience of serious illness, and how meeting another community member can be so intimate sometimes. There is nothing like that feeling of mutual understanding and empathy.

Ashley knocks on the door to Room 4 and then opens it. "Mr. Werner? I'm Ashley, the dietitian." She shakes his hand and then turns to his companions.

"I'm Elizabeth, his daughter," says the plump, white-haired lady sitting next to him. "And this is my husband, Tom."

"Nice to meet you all," says Ashley. "And this is Laura." She moves to the side and gestures at me.

"Hi!" I say brightly, shaking each person's hand. "I am a graduate student in communication, and I'm studying how staff and patients communicate together. Would it be okay if I listened while you talked with Ashley?" I scan Mr. Werner's face hopefully.

"Why, sure it would," says Mr. Werner, smiling broadly. Elizabeth nods and smiles too. Tom just sits stiffly.

I relax a bit. "Well, thank you very much." I lean against the counter and study Mr. Werner as Ashley explains the tasks she would complete with them. Always friendly and kind to patients, Ashley seems particularly gentle today.

Mr. Werner is quite short, not more than five foot or so. His broad face is lightly sun burned, and his blue eyes look intently at Ashley through his silver aviator glasses. The short sleeves of his light blue shirt expose ancient tattoos, smudged and sagging from the passing of time. My guess that he got them during military service is confirmed later on when he mentions being in the Navy to Elaine. The left leg of his black pants reveals the end of his metal prosthesis where his calf has been amputated. I feel a shiver go down my spine, and I look down at my own heavily scarred leg. It is hidden beneath the folds of my long, charcoal gray skirt, the outline of the plastic leg brace just visible beneath the soft flowing fabric. *Should I tell him?*

I tune back into the conversation as Ashley says, "Well, you should be eating a few more fruits and vegetables, but I am not going to try to change your eating habits after all these years." She smiles at him as she says this, and he nods.

"I eat well. I know because I do all the cooking!" says Mr. Werner with a smile.

Ashley chuckles. "You're doing just fine. I bet you are a good cook. Now I just need to measure your calf and your upper arm. This is a rough measure of your protein stores."

Smiling, Mr. Werner raises his left leg so the steel of the prosthesis catches the fluorescent light and shines. "How about measuring this one?" he jokes. We all laugh. Elizabeth looks at her father fondly. I laugh to avoid crying. Mr. Werner's cheerfulness seems sincere, but there also seems to be an undercurrent of sadness beneath it, unsurprisingly. I wish I could do something to help, something to give this kind man more time. As usual, there is nothing I can do. After over 2 years of not being able to do anything, I am becoming more resentful of my powerlessness, not less.

Ashley sits back down on her stool and records her measurements. "Do any of you have any questions for me?" she asks.

"No, I don't think so. Thank you," says Mr. Werner.

"OK, well here is my card. Feel free to call me if you think of anything later." Ashley stands up and shakes Mr. Werner's hand again. "It was nice to meet you," she says. Turning to his daughter and son-in-law, she adds, "Nice to meet you too."

"Thank you," says Elizabeth. Tom nods.

I step forward and smile. "I'll come back in with the next person, if that's all right with you?"

"Of course!" says Mr. Werner.

"Great," I say. Ashley walks out of the room, but I pause when I reach the door and look back. "You know," I say. "I have a confession. I wanted to meet you because I had a form of sarcoma that is very similar to the one you have."

"Really?" exclaims Mr. Werner in surprise.

I move closer to Mr. Werner and raise the right side of my skirt to reveal my bright blue plastic leg brace, purple scars, and grayish skin and muscle grafts.

"Wow!" he says. Elizabeth and Tom look at me eagerly.

"When did you have it?" asks Elizabeth.

"Ten years ago," I say. "It was really difficult." Understatement of the century.

Mr. Werner has tears in his eyes. "Did you have chemotherapy and surgery?"

"Yes, both," I say. I go on to explain the intricacies of my leg reconstruction and other treatments, adding that now I have severe osteoarthritis in my rebuilt knee.

"Wow," says Mr. Werner. "Well, that gives me some hope, since you survived."

"Well," I say. "It is *always* good to have hope." I want to cry because there is little hope of recovery for this warm and gentle stranger.

"Can I ask you something?" asks Mr. Werner tentatively.

"Of course," I say sincerely. "Anything."

"When you were sick and going through all the treatment, did you ever ask why me?" He looks at me, fear and fatigue in his eyes, and something else as well. Guilt, maybe?

"All the time," I answer honestly, my heart aching in my chest. Mr. Werner nods and I continue. "I asked that a lot. And I think it is an OK thing to do, I really believe that. You know, I still do some days. It's just that, well, at some point you have to move from 'why me?' to 'what am I going to do about it?' I mean, you can kind of go back and forth, acknowledging how awful and unfair it is, but then setting it aside and concentrating on living every day and trying to get well." I stop, not knowing what else to say, or even whether I have made any sense at all. "I'm just rambling, but. . . ."

"No," says Mr. Werner. "You're right. It's just . . . hard."

"Yes," I say, "It sure is." Our gazes lock for a moment, and I want to reach out and hug this man I have just met, but to whom I feel so connected. I don't. Instead, I tell him I will be right back when the doctor comes in.

"Sure," he says quietly. "I'll see you then." He manages a smile, and I smile back weakly before leaving.

I find Ashley and Joyce in the desk area and approach them. "I just feel so badly for Mr. Werner," I say.

"Me too," says Ashley.

"We all do," says Joyce. "I don't really think there is anything that can be done for him."

Nothing? We have been witnesses to his pain this morning. We have extended sympathy, listened attentively, offered information. That is something. I have to believe that is *something*. The team members must believe that too, or they could not come in and do their jobs every day.

I continue to observe and talk with the team members as they meet with Mr. Werner and the other patients in the clinic that day. Like an intricate but improvised dance, the process of moving back and forth through the door that separates the backstage staff area from the examination rooms reflects well-worn patterns of interaction while incorporating unique twists and turns in response to communication with both individual patients and other team members. I think back to the readings assigned in my health communication class. Although they gave me a good understanding of health care provider–patient communication and some understanding of professional communication within health care organizations, none of them explained what I was witnessing now. None of them theorized communication with patients and communication among health care professionals as being intimately connected in a reflexive relationship. Because it took me 2 years of observation to really develop my ideas about how the backstage and front stage communication produce each other, I am not surprised that few researchers have ventured into this world. Although researchers such as Putnam (1994) have long called for research on bona fide groups in natural (i.e., not researcher-constructed) settings, researchers eager to control variables and conditions find real teams messy to work with.

Ethnography is a method particularly well suited to such messy interaction, I think to myself as I walk to my car after 3 hours in the clinic have passed and I have surrendered to exhaustion. I slide my leg into the driver's seat of my sport coupe carefully, endeavoring to avoid putting any torque on my knee as I position myself behind the wheel, still thinking about mess. Not wanting to think anymore, I select CD #7 from my CD changer, an Indigo Girls' live album, and I belt out off-key renditions of their songs as I struggle through the congestion on the interstate.

I smile gratefully when I finally turn into my driveway; my husband's tiny blue Miata is already parked there. Gathering up my purse, the heavy canvas bag that holds my audio equipment and reading materials, my travel mug with the spicy-sweet remnants of my morning dose of chai, and my keys, I slam my car door. After struggling with the lock for a moment, I enter the house and unceremoniously drop all my stuff on the wide-shelved book-case in the entryway. Glenn comes out of his office to greet me.

"Hi, sweetie!" he says happily.

Folding myself into his arms, I murmur "Hi" into his shoulder and hold onto him tightly, letting the warmth of his body slowly soothe my raw nerves and aching heart as he lightly strokes my back. Glenn does not press me for an explanation; he is getting used to the way I come home from the clinic.

TASTE

I search frantically among my pillows and throw blankets for the dull pink basin. I can feel my stomach contracting, and within seconds I taste vomit as it spews up my throat. I grab the basin just in time to catch what had been my scant breakfast. The sour taste in my mouth lessens, but does not go away as I rinse again and again with seltzer water. Whenever I have surgery and am prescribed narcotics, I have the happy choice between pain or vom-iting because I have yet to find a narcotic that does not make me horribly nauseated. This knee replacement surgery is no exception—the pain is terri-ble, and so is the nausea. For now, I am vomiting; when the pain lessens a bit more, I will stop the medication.

I have been home from the hospital for just 3 days, following the surgery that attached an artificial knee joint to the bone graft that had replaced much of my femur years ago, and I am miserable. Glenn has gone back to work, and I am propped up on the couch for the day with an array of books and magazines, the TV remote, my laptop computer, printed drafts of sections of my manuscript, several bottles of medications, and a can of Canada Dry raspberry seltzer. As I take another swig of the fizzy water, I wish the pain and nausea were over for now. Of course they always come back.

It is early in my fieldwork, and I observe Dr. Armani as he talks with an unpleasant patient. The patient is a very large woman in her early 70s. An oxygen tube threads its way behind her ears and under her nose. Mrs. O'Neil wears a sleeveless hot pink blouse and clashing mauve vest and pants. Folds of fat hang loosely off her arms. Her enormous left breast, swollen from an inoperable tumor, droops down over her waist, straining taut the fabric of her blouse. Coarse white hair emerges from her scalp, abruptly turning bright dyed-orange after an inch or so. Dr. Armani begins to examine Mrs. O'Neil in preparation for her chemotherapy treatment in the infusion center down the hall.

On first sight of this woman sitting by her husband and young grandson, I feel only a distant and impersonal sympathy. I listen to her recount test results and symptoms to the doctor in her heavy Brooklyn accent, not unmoved by her plight, but tired and distracted by how much my knee hurts. I look up as Dr. Armani jumps up from his stool and takes Mrs. O'Neil's hand.

Mrs. O'Neil says simply, "Oh, and I had an endoscopy, did you get the results?" Abruptly I struggle to retain my composure as the force of my memory hits me. Ten years ago, I had an endoscopy.

"Swallow it. Swallow it," the technician insisted as he pushed the hard rubber tube deeper into my mouth. The command to swallow the inch-wide endoscopy tube seemed absurd—it could not possibly fit. "Swallow it. Come on, swallow it," he repeated. I gagged and vomited as he pushed the tube firmly to the very back of my mouth. Undeterred, the technician continued to push the tube until I swallowed it involuntarily. "Good," he said.

I felt pain and pressure as he forced the tube down my esophagus. A tiny camera documented each millimeter of the journey. I struggled to breathe while crying and vomiting continuously. Wave after wave of gagging hit me in rapid succession. I tried to breathe, tried to get away from the tube, but it moved with me as I dragged my head a few inches along the pillow. I sucked loud breaths, through my hose, unable to get enough air. Tears streamed out of my eyes and ran onto the white pillow case and sheet of the gurney on which I lay with my head turned to the right. Through my teary eyelashes, I saw a TV screen that displayed the camera's view of my esophagus. Two huge red sores glistened on the screen, the reason for this procedure.

The vomiting would not stop even though my stomach was empty. I concentrated on breathing and tried to stave off feelings of panic. The small dose of Valium the technician had given me made me a bit groggy, but could not dull the sensation of suffocating. *I can't breathe*, I screamed silently. *Make it stop! Take it out!* My eyes implored the nurse who held my hand. She looked at me with compassion in her eyes and said, "It's almost over." The dry heaves were still coming fast, without interruption—heave . . . heave . . . heave . . . *Make it stop!*

Oblivious to me, the technician continued to look at the sores with interest.

Abruptly, I jerk myself back to the interaction in Mrs. O'Neil's examination room. I taste bile, gag, and quickly try to cover it up by coughing. I do not want Mrs. O'Neil to think she is the cause of my gagging. My stomach churns, and I tremble silently as I try to shake away the memory that burst through to my consciousness when Mrs. O'Neil spoke the word, endoscopy. I look at the woman with a new compassion, the memory of the horror of the procedure moving me almost to tears on behalf of us both.

* * *

Memories of vomit crowd my mind and worsen my nausea, so I munch a cracker and try to think of far more pleasant times when eating was a pleasure instead of a precarious effort to get something to stay down. In my mind, I can taste the four-cheese pizza from the IOPOA Christmas party from 3 months ago.

The pizza was a masterful blend of tastes and textures, piping hot, and redolent of Parmesan cheese and basil. As they put it on the table in front of us, I smiled at Ashley, Elaine's husband Bill, and Lin Su, a graduate student from the Aging Studies department who conducts research with the IOPOA. We sat together on high stools at a table in the upstairs bar area of a local brew pub. It was late January, and the team was just now having its holiday celebration, having been unable to find a good time for everyone in the rush of the holidays. Like their team meetings, retreats, and so many other functions, the IOPOA party was sponsored by a pharmaceutical company whose representative cheerfully presided over the casual gathering. Ashley's boyfriend was playing pool with Beth's husband and some other patrons of the bar. Groups of two, three, or four clustered, cheerfully chatting and joking while sipping an array of microbrews produced on the premises.

As we eat four-cheese pizza together, we pull slices from the silver pan, and I smile to myself as it occurs to me that, in a way, sharing a pizza is the modern equivalent of the ancient practice of breaking bread together. In sharing this meal and the lively conversation, I get a taste of what their lives are like outside of the clinic and conference room walls. We sample a wide range of topics.

Intrigued by the memory of that night at the brewery, I open my laptop and make some notes in the chapter 4 file. Thinking of pizza is not helping my churning stomach at all, so I try to think about other things for awhile as I chew a couple of Tums, their chalky taste slightly dulling the bitterness of bile. My thoughts wander, and I review the 5 days spent in the cancer center with my knee replacement surgery. Images of pain and vomit and late-night loneliness surface. Abruptly I remember a particular incident that occurred on the second day of my admission, when two parts of my life collided with each other.

I woke up groggily at the knock on my hospital room door. Suppressing a groan, I called out, "Yes?"

Three young people in lab coats entered, two women and a man. "We're your pain team," said the man exuberantly, as if he felt sure I would be delighted with this news. I felt disgusting—my unwashed hair hung in limp tangles on my shoulders, yellow splotches of Betadyne, necessitated by my allergy to surface alcohol, were scattered over my arms from several attempts to start an IV, nausea reeled in my stomach, the taste of bile lingered in my mouth—and the last thing I wanted was to talk to anymore medical personnel. I smiled in what I hoped was a friendly manner as they introduced themselves. As I looked from one to the other, I suddenly realized that one of the woman on the team was a pharmacy resident whom I had seen in several team meetings as she shadowed Susan, the IOPOA team pharmacist. Her name was Marcy; she recognized me too.

"Oh—hi!" said Marcy, surprised recognition crossing her face.

"Hi. You work with Susan, right?" I asked, just to be sure.

"Yes, I did. I am on the pain team rotation now," she said calmly. "Nice to see you."

A sickening sense of shame washed over me. I hated being seen as a patient by anyone associated with the IOPOA team. Although all the team members were aware of my past experience with cancer and had seen my impaired and disfigured leg, none of them had actually seen me in a hospital bed, wearing a gown, with an IV in my arm.

The pain team visit was interrupted by the appearance of a young man with a stretcher. "I have to take you down to x-ray," he said simply.

"We'll come back," said the male resident on the team whose name I had not paid attention to, as the three of them turned and walked out of my room.

Not two minutes later, as the young man pushed me down the hall, I saw Ashley, the team dietitian, standing by the nurse's station. She looked attractive and professional in a blue flowered dress and her customary white coat.

"Hi, Laura," she said cheerfully.

"Oh, hi!" I said, the shame returning in full force. Laying on the stretcher, I was conscious of my inability to stand up, to stop the man from continuing to push me down the hall, to even approximate the role of a professional.

"How are you feeling?" Ashley inquired kindly, walking along side me, her hand resting lightly on the rail of the stretcher.

"Oh, I'm hanging in there," I said with as much cheerfulness as I could manage.

"Hope you're feeling better," she said, stopping as we boarded the elevator.

"Thanks. See you later," I called out as the doors shut behind me. Tears of frustration and helplessness pricked at the corners of my eyes.

Shaking my head over this memory, I wonder whether Ashley had felt uncomfortable witnessing me playing a very different role than the one with which she was accustomed. Two parts of my life had come in contact, two roles I was usually able to keep sharply distinct from one another, and I felt like a failure. When the two roles had collided, the carefully managed persona of a competent communication researcher had been immediately and totally eclipsed by the role of the patient.

*　*　*

A month later, I am getting around on crutches, off the narcotics, and feeling a lot better. I bustle around the kitchen preparing a snack for Sandra and me. As Sandra bounces her 8-month-old son, David, on her knee, I serve lemonade and gingersnaps one-handedly, returning to the kitchen from the adjacent dining room four times while balancing on one crutch and carrying in the other hand, in turn, two tall glasses, a plate of cookies, and a handful of napkins.

"Can't I give you hand?" asks Sandra sweetly. "I can put him down."

"No, no. I can do it," I respond, stubbornly refusing to take anymore help than I absolutely need. I smile, determined to be a good host. Sandra has come to let me interview her and solicit her feedback on my preliminary findings. Satisfied that everything is on the table, I nod and then ease myself into a chair, leaning my crutch against the wall behind me.

"He is getting so big!" I say, gazing with some longing at the beautiful baby.

"I know," says Sandra, shaking her head. She takes a sip of her lemonade. "He's such a little man now—he really wants to crawl, you can see it on his face."

I take a ginger snap and savor the first bite. We begin talking about the clinic, and I ask for her reaction to the table in which I have carefully delineated seven backstage communicative processes. "Feel free to criticize or disagree with it," I add, just in case.

"Yes, you've got it, you do, only—" She pauses. "It's just that it doesn't happen one at a time. It is controlled chaos. And yet that chaos works. Most of the time it works really well. It just sort of happens and then at the end I was left to assemble a story that reflected all that we had found about each patient." Sandra looks thoughtful and I nod encouragingly. She pauses and nibbles a cookie.

"The way I have separated out the different forms of communication for discussion makes it sound as if it is a more orderly process than it really is," I say, nodding.

"Yes," says Sandra. "When we started out, Dr. Armani and I, we had an idea of how it would work, but we really didn't know what would happen. This system just sort of developed as we went along. And some people work better together than others, and some days it seems like we aren't communicating and nothing is working at all. But most of the time, it works. And it works really well."

"It sure does," I agree, nodding.

"And it was me, and now Elaine, who had to pull it all together, to do the dictation and try to make sense of it all, to create a story of the patient's visit *as a whole*." She looks thoughtful and I nod silently, waiting for her to go on.

"It's all a process of making sense of all the little bits of the data, of the patient, of putting it all together," said Sandra.

"So the information sharing and the other things that happen in the backstage, those weren't decided on ahead of time when the team was designed?"

"No, not at all. We were winging it. We still are, really," she concludes.

"Me too," I respond.

* * *

After Sandra leaves, I sit down on my couch and flip on Food TV network for background noise. "East Meets West with Ming Tsai" is on, I note happily. It is one of the better shows on this season. As Ming starts making nouveau sushi, I open my cute blue iBook laptop, a bribe from myself and my husband to motivate me to finish my manuscript. I am feeling wounded and worried. I have written stories and written analysis. I have written reflections, and I have written what Laurel Richardson (2000) called "writing-stories"—stories about the process of writing. I keep trying to figure out how to blend more than one form of writing. Moreover, I am completely overwhelmed by the amount of data I have gathered; I have several books worth of material. At the same time, I know that I could learn so much more if I continued to spend time with the IOPOA team.

I want to give my readers a taste of how the IOPOA looks, feels, sounds, and smells. I want to show *and* tell. I sample different writing strategies, trying to find one that will work, but no single genre allows me to accomplish all of my objectives. I question the wisdom of offering competing perspectives, a melange of flavors and textures that contrast pleasingly with each other, while harmonizing around a central theme. I look up from my computer, still unsure what to do. Checking back in with Ming Tsai, I see that he is mixing wasabi powder and canola oil into a thick paste. As he arranges little tidbits of sushi on a platter, it occurs to me that I am offering up my findings buffet style, inviting the reader to a little of this and a little of that, a range of tastes, but not a lot of any single one. A lover of dim sum, wine and cheese tastings, and Sunday brunch buffets, I am drawn to bits and pieces, artfully arranged to please the eye and the palate. I know that readers more accustomed to being served results in one genre are unlikely to feel satisfied by my offerings. However, perhaps it is good that I am disrupting their expectations.

In the introduction to *Women Writing Culture*, Behar (1995) noted that feminists undermine their own credibility in the (already skeptical) eyes of the positivists and postpositivists who still populate the academy when they express doubt about their fieldwork or writing practices. Yet Behar believes that self-scrutiny and revealing the constructed nature of knowledge production is essential, as do other feminist theorists such as Haraway (1988). This self-doubt threatens to overwhelm my ability to write, yet this doubt is part of being an ethnographer. Why is it that the less powerful are willing to own up to the doubt? What do I gain by not only admitting my doubts, but consciously and deliberately drawing attention to them by mixing writing forms and arguing that the forms both support *and* subvert each other, reinforce *and* undermine existing power structures, and reflect my privilege *and* my marginalization? What do I lose?

POWER: A SIXTH SENSE

> Connecting and writing lives is also about connecting and writing about the embodiedness and physicality of the self. The peopling of biography and ethnography is physical as well as social and cultural. In writing ethnography, we are engaged in a practice of writing and rewriting the body. (Coffey, 1999, p. 131)

A cartoon recently cut from *The New Yorker* marks my place in *Women Writing Culture*. Flipping open the book, I stare at the caricature of author Stephen King—who recently survived being hit by a van—in a bathrobe and striped pajamas. He supports his body with two red crutches that morph into fountain pens at the bottom. From the tips of both pen/crutches, words flow freely, looping up to surround his body.

I cut the image out of the magazine because it reminds me that from experiencing and witnessing pain, recovery, and loss, writing is born. Writing comes from the body, inscribes the body, heals the body. At the same time, in the writing, other bodies are inscribed—perhaps healed, perhaps wounded, more likely both. As I have written the bodies of the team members, other clinic staff members, patients, patients' companions, and, of course, myself, I have chosen some details and omitted far more. I have inscribed meanings related to illness, age, race, gender, and a host of other individual and social factors.

Starhawk (1988) reminded us that we do not have to always think of power as dominating or having control over others. There is also generative power, what she called "immanent power," power from within that can be a positive force in the world.

> When we plant, when we weave, *when we write*, when we give birth, when we organize, when we heal, when we run through the park while the redwoods sweat mist, when we do what we're afraid to do, we are not separate. We are of the world and of each other, and the power within us is a great, if not invincible power. Though we can be hurt, we can heal; though each one of us can be destroyed, within us is the power of renewal. And there is still time to choose that power. (p. 14; italics added)

As I struggle to write ethnography and analysis, I choose the immanent power of writing, hoping that writing will help bring about healing for patients, their companions, the team members, and myself.

5

———◆———

COMMUNICATING
POWER

Teamwork is inextricably imbued with relations of power. . . . The
issue for teams is not to seek to avoid power but [to] recogniz[e]
how crucially it structures their work. (Opie, 2000, p. 255)

Illuminating the taken-for-granted power relations in which health care
teams work is a crucial first step toward promoting positive change in
processes in which communication is stymied by unproductive use of power
and further enhancing effective communication. The three portrayals of
teamwork in the preceding chapters each shed light on particular aspects of
the team's communication in the clinic. Yet all of them leave largely unquestioned the system in which communication patterns were developed, negotiated, maintained, and modified. The seven backstage processes explicated
in the grounded theory analysis and reflected in the narrative ethnography
and autoethnography were heavily constrained by, and must be situated
within, the team's immediate context—the cancer center—and the larger
context of the U.S. medical establishment.

Because a major motivation for the use of interdisciplinary teams in health care settings is to enable close collaboration across disciplinary lines (e.g., Opie, 2000) and to provide high-quality care to patients (Rubenstein et al., 1991), the manner in which medical establishment norms of hierarchy constrained the team members' backstage communication is critical to understanding teamwork effectiveness. Medical care is deeply divided along disciplines, and a rigid hierarchy of disciplinary power tends to characterize hospitals and clinics, reinforcing physician power as natural and inevitable while marginalizing members of less powerful disciplines (Wear, 1997). Teams are usually intended to promote egalitarian interactions; however, they often maintain professional hierarchies far more than they subvert them (Cott, 1998). Moreover, the issue for theorists of teamwork is not that power disparities exist among disciplines and among demographic groups, but

> how the relations of (disciplinary) power existing in a particular team affect how the team as a team elicits and engages with information from its different disciplinary sites and how, as a result of including or marginalizing particular types of knowledge, a specific team inscribes the bodies of its clients/families and itself, a process with material outcomes for all of the three groups involved. (Opie, 2000, p. 255)

That is, power makes some voices heard and silences or diminishes others, heavily influencing what knowledge goes into the IOPOA team's construction of a comprehensive assessment and treatment plan for each patient and patients' engagement (or lack thereof) with that plan.

To some readers, my attention to power may seem abstract or tangential to understanding the daily task of providing and receiving health care. I illustrate the pervasiveness of power through a brief example. Consider the following backstage interaction:

> "This patient is a true Southern pain-in-the-ass," declares IOPOA nurse practitioner, Sandra Bates, as she approaches the desk to report to Dr. Armani, the oncologist who directs the IOPOA. I chuckle at the image. Sandra continues, "She has all this information her daughter got off the Internet and she is refusing to have her chemotherapy treatment until Dr. Armani explains to her the justification for her protocol. She wouldn't accept my explanation; she wants 'the doctor.'" Sandra shakes her head in frustration.
>
> Dr. Armani sighs in exasperation. "These patients who get on the Internet, they never get enough information to understand their situation, just enough to cause problems. They argue with me but don't understand what they are arguing about."

As the team members talk, I recall a study that reported that patients who insisted on asking questions and discussing treatment options were labeled "difficult," and physicians complained that such patients wasted too much of their time. I believe that patient education and self-advocacy can be very beneficial, but I remain silent.

In this brief exchange, power is invoked but taken for granted by Sandra, Dr. Armani, myself, and the patient. Power was manifested in (at least) the following 10 ways:

◀ The patient claimed informational/knowledge power based on the medical research she had gathered.

◀ The nurse practitioner used her own power to attempt to thwart the patient's claim to informational power by offering her a placating explanation.

◀ The patient asserted her power by resisting the nurse practitioner's authority and demanding to speak with the physician.

◀ The nurse practitioner used her professional and institutional power to leave the examination room (in which the patient was confined) to go to the backstage space and engage in cathartic venting to sympathetic colleagues.

◀ The physician and nurse practitioner marginalized the patients' voice and dismissed both her claim to specific treatment-related knowledge and her claim of her capacity to produce knowledge at all ("they *never* get enough information to understand . . . ").

◀ The nurse practitioner acknowledged that handling the patient would take more power than she had and enlisted the physicianís authority to gain patient compliance.

◀ The physician accepted as natural that his power was greater than the nurse practitioner's, and he did not attempt to empower her to resolve the problem herself.

◀ As a researcher, I complied with the institutional and professional power of the physician and nurse practitioner by refusing to intervene and allowing them to assume that I agreed with their expressed views on patient self-education.

◀ I invoked disciplinary power as a communication researcher/scholar by labeling the patient "difficult" using the criteria I garnered from health communication research.

◀ The physician reinforced physician power and participated in the undermining of nurse practitioner power and of patient power by explaining the treatment protocol to the patient without confronting the patient's rejection of the nurse practitioner's knowledge or acknowledging the patient's own ability to construct knowledge.

Clearly, power was operating on multiple levels throughout this interaction. Regardless of whether these power relations are beneficial or harmful, they must be acknowledged. I seek not to blame anyone, but to point out how power is operating so that we as scholars and practitioners can reflect on how power enhances and/or detracts from our goals of studying and improving communication for the benefit of everyone involved in the system. I offer here a rich description of how power operates, but I have resisted the temptation to provide tidy solutions to the problems I explore.

I offer some concrete implications and practical suggestions for administrators and team members in chapter 6, but I cannot offer any fail-proof formulas or techniques for coping with the complex problems relating to power differences that health care teams face. Teams are embedded within overlapping webs of power—institutional, cultural, political, professional, social, and individual. Addressing one aspect of power cannot release a team from the rest of the intricately woven webs surrounding them. Thus, it can be frustrating to become aware of just how imbued with power everyday health care interactions are, and that frustration can turn to defensiveness, anger, or hopelessness. My goal in promoting awareness of power is not to frustrate readers, but to provide them with a perspective that they can draw on when making choices about how to respond when faced with opportunities for communication, which is what Stewart and Logan (1998) called "nexting"—the ability to choose to respond fruitfully, helpfully, and positively regardless of how negative the communication may be to which you are responding. Although the particular circumstances of the IOPOA team members are unique, health care teams in any institutional context face similar challenges.

In this chapter, I explore some of the myriad of ways in which power manifests itself in daily clinical practice and the researching thereof. To situate this discussion, I provide a brief history of the modern medical profession. Then I extend Opie's (2000) insightful work on power and knowledge construction in team meetings by exploring how power manifests itself in backstage communication within the clinic, with particular attention to the naturalization of physician power and the ambivalence surrounding nurse practitioner power. Next, I explore how frontstage communication between team members and patients reflects and reinforces disciplinary power differences among team members and between health care professionals and patients. Finally, I explore how my research process has both resisted and supported the power hierarchy within the IOPOA team and the medical system in general.

HISTORICAL CONTEXT OF THE U.S. MEDICAL ESTABLISHMENT

To understand the power dynamics that play out in day-to-day communication among team members, it is helpful to have a cursory understanding of the ways in which the modern practice of medicine developed over the previous 150 years. After reviewing that history, I explore briefly the nature of large bureaucratic institutions, of which the medical establishment is arguably the most socially and politically powerful in contemporary U.S. society (Gürsoy, 1996; Williams & Calnan, 1996; Zola, 1990). I am not describing the evolution of physicians' power in order to bash physicians or demonize the American Medical Association (AMA). My goal is to explore the possibilities for a medical system that is more humane to both practitioners and patients, and I cannot do so without first describing how power is currently manifested and how it came to be that way.

The current U.S. medical system is neither natural nor neutral; it is the result of specific historical events, and it affords more power to some individuals and groups than others (Ehrenreich & English, 1973; Foucault, 1973/1994). Power in the medical academy involves complex contemporary and historical intersections of race, gender, class, sexuality, educational level, and able-bodied privilege and oppressions (Wear, 1997). The U.S. system of health care delivery as it currently exists is the culmination of a series of historical events, as well as the adaptations that continue in light of recent events and innovations. Respect for physician authority remains quite high despite recent trends toward a more consumerist mindset on the part of some patients who seek decision-making power in their health care (e.g., Roter, Stewart, Putnam, Lipkin, Stiles, & Inui, 1997). The prestige and authority afforded physicians in the U.S. has its roots in late 19th- and early 20th-century efforts to professionalize the field of medicine and transform it from folk medicine, "barber surgeon," and religious or faith healing traditions into a scientific practice that relied on rigorous research and increasingly sophisticated diagnostic technologies (du Pre, 1999). The 1910 Flexner Report, commissioned by the AMA, harshly criticized medical school curriculum and training and led to the eventual closing of nearly two thirds of all U.S. medical schools, as well as major reform within the remaining schools. As part of their professionalization efforts, the AMA launched a campaign to discredit folk healers, midwives, and other "alternative" practitioners. Lobbying by the AMA led to outlawing many dangerous and unproven practices (as well as some beneficial ones such as midwifery, unfortunately), standardization of training, and licensing of physicians. Physicians' authority, bolstered by their extensive training, use of technology, and adherence to scientific research principles, became widely accepted, and physicians' expertise was considered virtually unquestionable (du Pre, 1999). Home visits ceased, and medical care became centralized in hospitals and clinics where technology was readily available and numerous patients could be seen more efficiently. At the same time that physician prestige and authority increased, their responsibility and liability increased; as the top of the medical hierarchy, physicians are held accountable for malpractice claims.

The history of medical care shapes its current norms, along with more recent issues, such as extensive specialization, spiraling medical costs, widespread implementation of managed care systems, increasing need for chronic illness management (rather than curing), and resurgent interest by patients in alternative and complementary medicine (Geist-Martin, Ray, & Sharf, 2003). Social forces affect the patterns of communication that emerge in clinical interaction, specifically physician dominance and patient submission to authority. Despite the advent of dramatic changes such as managed care, physicians remain highly respected, well paid (although less so than before managed care), and very powerful both within health care organizations and in society at large (e.g., Frank, 1995). Thus, the medical clinic context is not merely the background in which IOPOA backstage team communication processes developed and are continually negotiated. On the contrary, the present (and historic) conditions of the medical system, to a great degree, *gave rise to the communicative processes* described in this book. The Western medical context in which the team operated is not an objective factor existing outside of the group; it is enacted through language in team members' daily communication with each other (Barge & Keyton, 1994).

The medical establishment, like all institutional power systems, obscures its socially constructed nature, making it appear natural, inevitable, and normal; it produces standards for evaluation and then justifies itself according to those standards (Foucault, 1975/1995). Bureaucracies such as Western medical systems, particularly the U.S. capitalistic incarnation, have as their primary goal conservation—their continued existence; all other functions support the primary goal (Ferguson, 1984). Such systems privilege particular groups (and their values, culture, language, and modes of behavior) over others while obscuring (through language) that privilege as inevitable and normative. Moreover, when members of traditionally less powerful groups move into more powerful institutional positions, they tend to adopt many of the values and norms of the groups that traditionally held power over them, and little or no systemic change occurs (Wear, 1997).

Using the standards established by the medical system, the communication processes that I described in the narratives and in the analysis seemed to work well overall and be fairly unproblematic. Physician authority over other health care providers, for example, seems to be an efficient and effective model for clinical practice, as evidenced by the fact that the team does a good job providing care to their patients. The system becomes self-justifying—having made up the norms and standards for what medical care is and how it should be provided and received, the medical system then evaluates itself (and invites others evaluate it) using only those same (socially constructed) norms and standards. Needing help, patients are often afraid, and they buy into the worldview that is necessary to get medical care; even when displeased, we still tend to think within existing systemic constraints as if they were inevitable. Likewise, researchers of health care settings tend to take for granted many aspects of the system as unchangeable even when these aspects have significant negative impacts.

COMMUNICATING DIVERSITY AND POWER

———

Liberal feminists in the 1980s initially placed their hope in the "critical mass" approach to creating a more egalitarian system; that is, once enough women were physicians, the medical system would become less hierarchical and more egalitarian in its values and communication styles. That has not been the case; despite equal numbers of women and men and increasing percentages of people of color being admitted to medical schools, the power has not shifted. Positions in the highest levels of medicine are still largely held by White men, and the few members of other groups who make it into high levels of medicine tend to reflect the same traditional values[1] (Wear, 1997). Biological sex of doctors is now more equally distributed; however, the gendered nature of roles within medical care has remained largely static. That is, although women are physicians, the role of a physician remains vested with masculine power. Likewise, a small but increasing number of nurses are men (5.4%, according to the Bureau of Health Professions 2001, cited in www.NurseZone.com), but the role remains feminine because of its long association with women and submission of (female) nurses to (male) physicians (Allen, 1997; Prescott & Bowen, 1985).[2] Because those in power are

———

[1]The perpetuation of male privilege, power, and bias in medicine also is due, at least in part, to the fact that the overwhelming majority of administrative positions in medical schools remains the exclusive purview of White men. For example, despite that women make up fully half of all incoming medical students, only 4 of the 127 medical schools in the United States are headed by a woman dean; the number of woman full professors averages 16 per medical school, compared with 155 men per school; very few department chairs in medical schools are women (Wear, 1997); and the American Medical Association (AMA) has had only one female executive officer in its 144-year history, elected in 1998 (du Pre, 1999). Furthermore, the medical academy is overwhelmingly White and upper middle class in background, and the higher levels of medical administration are made up primarily of people of European descent (Wear, 1997). Women of color are overrepresented among the lowest paid health care workers, who primarily do direct, hands-on care (Sacks, 1988).

[2]One study reported that 55% of nurses surveyed found working with female physicians to be no better or worse than working with male physicians (Nursing 91, 1991). This may be because female physicians are trained largely by men according to masculine norms (Northrup, 1994; Wear, 1997).

responsible for training the next generation of physicians, traditional values and norms are passed on through language with minimal changes regardless of the demographic makeup of the incoming class of medical students. Those changes that are made occur well within the context (language and taken-for-granted parameters) of the existing systems of power (as does this book, for the most part).

Physicians remain firmly ensconced as team leaders (a physician directs the IOPOA) and administrators, with the majority of the high-ranking physicians on teams being men and the vast majority of the lower status professions represented on health care teams (e.g., nurses and social workers) being women, including women of color (Cowen, 1992; Fagin, 1992; Wear, 1997). The power disparity can cause a great deal of resentment and impede successful collaboration efforts (Abramson & Mizrahi, 1996; Fagin, 1992; Iles & Auluck, 1990; Lichtenstein et al., 1997). Perceptions of teamwork effectiveness vary significantly between the highly prestigious, highly paid positions of physician and administrator, and the relatively low ranking positions of some team members, such as nurses and other direct caregivers (Berteotti & Seibold, 1994; Cott, 1998; Griffiths, 1998). Thus, the effectiveness of teams may be tempered through their privileging some members' voices over others. Given the stratification in medical institutions, communication with a team is likely to be, at least in part, a function of its members' relative power within the medical hierarchy and often their gender and cultural backgrounds, which tend to correlate with traditional social hierarchies.

The membership of the IOPOA team largely mirrors historical gender and racial hierarchies in health care, with some important exceptions. Yet analysis of the team members' gender, sexuality, class, and cultural identities does not reveal the complexity of their interactions and the systems of power that underlie them. An argument could be made for the cultural diversity of the team, and an equally compelling one could be made for homogeneity of the team. The IOPOA team could be thought of as diverse particularly because of the arrival of the second nurse practitioner. The team was entirely White when I began this project. The second nurse practitioner is Cuban American; she is bilingual, speaking English without a Latin accent and fluent Spanish. Both the oncologists immigrated to the United States from Europe; the director, Dr. Armani, is from Italy, and Dr. Klein is from Switzerland. Both speak English with pronounced European accents. Moreover, Dr. Klein is a female oncologist, which breaks the cultural stereotype of male physicians—a stereotype that is challenged increasingly by women specialists (at this writing, the president of the American Society of Clinical Oncology is a woman), but remains deeply ingrained in public consciousness.

However, the relative homogeneity of the team is also easy to establish. Of the 12 team members (due to staff turnover during my fieldwork) with whom I spent time in the clinic, 9 were White middle-class women raised in the United States (as am I). Most of the team members have attained a master's or higher level of education, and all have bachelor's degrees; I had two master's degrees during my fieldwork and have since completed my Ph.D. The oncologists were from Western Europe. Although they certainly have cultural experiences and beliefs not held by other team members or myself, their worldviews, as played out in clinic teamwork, reflected mainstream Euro-American norms of politeness, forms of address, and nonverbal signals such as eye contact. Moreover, the oncologists' practice of medicine largely reflected the Western model of medicine embraced by the cancer center and more generally in the U.S. medical establishment.[3] Also, although there was a female oncologist (occupying a powerful position traditionally occupied by men), there were no male professionals among the nonphysician team members (occupying less powerful positions traditionally occupied by women). The certified nursing assistants (those with the least power in the clinic)— who are not considered part of the team, but who perform services for the team in the clinic—were all African-American or Latina women without bachelor's degrees.

Middle- or upper class socioeconomic status (SES) was also part of the socially constructed world of the team. Team members' discussions of purchasing houses, high-quality clothes, cars, computers, and other expensive goods and services, and the lack of conversations about negotiating public transportation or coping with the bureaucracy of public assistance agencies, reaffirmed this unspoken norm. Likewise communication assumed normative heterosexuality, taking for granted (leaving unsaid) that people identified as heterosexual. Most of the team members were married or in heterosexual relationships. It is certainly possible that some members of the team were not heterosexual, but if so, those identities were not discussed or in any way referred to within my hearing in the clinic or team meetings. Discussions of marriage, childrearing, and dating all assumed heterosexuality by never mentioning it; through language, then, the team socially constructs norms that reinforce certain identities and marginalize others.

Thus, the issue is not that the team members engaged in racist, sexist, classist, or homophobic rhetoric as they communicated in the backstage, but that a team norm was jointly constructed as much by what was *not* said as by what was commented on openly. That norm reflects historical stereotypes far more than it calls them into question. Readers can decide for themselves whether the team qualifies as diverse, according to their pre-

---

[3]Dr. Armani's philosophy of medicine (and life) differed in important ways in terms of how he communicated with and treated patients; he appeared much more comfortable with discussing and accepting death, for example, than most other physicians I have encountered. However, his administration of the IOPOA team reflected norms similar to those of his U.S.-trained physician colleagues.

ferred criteria, or perhaps determine that it is impossible to judge based on the information I have provided. My point is that nothing about the team's collaboration represents a serious challenge to the prevailing power structures in Western medicine. The biologically female physician, for example, has not undone the masculine privilege associated with the physician role through the presence of her female body in that position of power; her femininity is cast as an exception to the rule. Likewise, there are no social workers giving orders to physicians. The issue is not that the IOPOA team has failed to diversify or reject the traditional forms of power into which they were socialized, but that *such power remains masked.* As long as power goes unnoted, it is naturalized. I do not want to minimize important changes that patients, health care providers, and other activists have worked for in health care organization and delivery. Yet I do want to point out that all of these changes (as reflected in the team that I have studied) function well within existing power structures and do not threaten radical (or even significant) change to the overarching systems of power that are perpetuated in late modern capitalistic medicine.

In the IOPOA, caring professionals work hard to deliver high quality care to their patients. Yet their daily clinical teamwork reproduces traditional power structures far more than it subverts them. At issue is not only the quality of care according to existing standards, but also the possibilities of care under other models and the physical, emotional, and social health of the health care and social service professionals who provide that care.[4] To begin to envision systemic change requires scholars, practitioners, patients, and patients' companions recognize the parameters of the system in which they are embedded. Marking taken-for-granted power through language is not a solution to what ails the U.S. medical system, but it is a necessary beginning. Likewise, marking the ways in which my production of this text invokes and reifies power hierarchies does not undo my complicity. However, in persevering in this project, I offer the hope that "the slight flapping of the wings of a feminist butterfly might—metaphorically—provide the trigger that would enable [the patriarchal system] to flip over into a state of radical change" (Battersby, 1999, p. 355).[5]

To that end, I explore several specific ways in which power is enacted, reinforced, and resisted in the backstage communicative processes of teamwork and in the relationship between these processes and team member communication with patients. I then explore the ways in which my research and writing practices reflect my own use of power.

---

[4]The rates of burnout and stress-related health conditions are very high among health care providers, especially physicians (e.g., Bonsteel, 1997; Pincus, 1995).

[5]Battersby (1999) is, of course, referring to a principle of chaos theory here; that " . . . something as slight as the flapping of a butterfly's wings in the Pacific might act as the trigger that 'causes' a hurricane on the other side of the world" (p. 351).

POWER IN CLINIC TEAMWORK

Perpetuation of Physician Privilege

Despite organizational attempts to encourage collaboration, physician power remains an unexamined axiom that provides the foundation for nonegalitarian teamwork (Berteotti & Seibold, 1994; Cott, 1998; Griffiths, 1998). The continued focus on the physician as the primary decision maker and his or her visit as the pinnacle of the team's interaction with the patient contributes to the privilege of physicians over the others in the perceptions of patients, patients' companions,[6] team members, and other clinic staff not affiliated with the IOPOA who share clinic space with the team (Abramson & Mizrahi, 1996; Cott, 1998; Fagin, 1992; Griffiths, 1998; Iles & Auluck, 1990; Lichtenstein et al., 1997). The team operated within an unspoken but persistent hierarchy of power despite what I perceived to be its collegiality and the genuine good will on the part of both oncologists. Listed in descending order, the team hierarchy, as I perceived it and as two team members articulated to me in interviews, was as follows: a physician was both director of the team and clinical oncologist who saw roughly two thirds of the IOPOA's patients; a second physician was head of the team's research program and clinical oncologist to approximately a third of the team's patients; a nurse practitioner saw all IOPOA patients, acted as information gatekeeper in the clinic, dictated clinic notes on behalf of both her and the oncologists, and facilitated team meetings; the dietitian, social worker, and pharmacist saw all IOPOA patients and produced their own clinic notes in addition to formally reporting key information to the nurse practitioner; and two registered nurses were each assigned to one of the oncologists and saw that oncologist's patients. At the very bottom of the hierarchy, nursing assistants recorded patients' vital signs for the team, but were not considered part of the team nor invited to collaborate; they were nonpersons involved in the team's performance, but generally ignored (Goffman, 1959). Other oncologists working within the clinic with the team functioned as equal in power to the team's oncologists.

---

[6]I have written elsewhere about the impact of the patients' companions on their interactions with the team members (Ellingson, 2002). Companions varied in their behavior with physicians, but many behaved in ways that reinforced the physician's higher status. Companions, for example, often asked each nonphysician team member when the doctor would be coming and whether they had to see anyone else before the doctor. Quite a few companions also appeared to take nonphysician staff less seriously, engaging in other tasks (e.g., reading) while other team members talked with patients, but giving the physician their full attention.

Moreover, racial and gender privilege intersected to reinforce oncologists' higher status within the clinic hierarchy, further widening the social divisions, enabling oncologists to assert their privilege, and encouraging others to accommodate their space management demands, albeit with some resentment (Wear, 1997). Unsurprisingly, three of the four oncologists I observed were men, and all were White; the nursing assistants and support staff were all female, and, of the five I observed, one was African American, one was White, and three were Latina. The second nurse practitioner I observed was Latina; all other team members and clinic personnel were White middle-class women. The exceptions to the traditional hierarchy (e.g., a female oncologist) were not sufficient to negate the tradition of power based on historical gender and racial disparities that formed an integral (although largely unacknowledged) aspect of the context in which space was negotiated (Ehrenreich & English, 1973; Wear, 1997). Additionally, although there were examples of lower status groups moving upward in the hierarchy (the female oncologist, the Latina nurse practitioner), there were no examples of men occupying lower status positions such as nursing assistant.

Awareness of this power hierarchy was reported in interviews with team members, and I observed its manifestation in many aspects of backstage communication. Next I discuss four particular ways in which hierarchy constrained backstage communication (see chap. 3 for a detailed discussion of backstage communication processes).

First, informal information and impression sharing, in which team members voluntary sought out one another for cross-disciplinary collaboration and boundary blurring, occurred primarily among team members of similar status level—dietitian, social worker, and pharmacist. The registered nurses, oncologists, and the nurse practitioner participated much less often. This finding relates to Cott's (1998) argument that team members tend to have different meanings for teamwork depending on their status. The dietitian, social worker, and pharmacist pooled information and impressions to accomplish specific objectives (e.g., the dietitian asked the pharmacist to reinforce a message about vitamin dosage to accomplish her specific dietary objective of persuading a patient not to overdose on a vitamin). The oncologists, in contrast, saw other team members as providing important screenings and information to the patients, and as providing the oncologists through formal reporting with an array of information that they could take into consideration as they made their treatment recommendations, but not as helping them with a given task.

These different understandings of teamwork correspond with levels of power, not just different roles. Informal information and impression sharing occurred most readily among those whose status similarities fostered comfortable boundary blurring; there was little social risk in the negotiation when all participants had roughly equal power and responsibility. The lack of informal cross-status collaboration reinforces power hierarchy by fostering blurring of roles only within a given level of power and leaving unquestioned each discipline's power. The existence of "fundamental social divisions" within the team and the clinic limited perceptions of backstage familiarity and informality among members of different groups (Goffman, 1959). Although Goffman suggests that mutual dependence on fellow team members to carry out the frontstage performance fosters cohesion among team members, this is clearly a case in which a socially constructed division based on prestige and power limited the degree of cohesiveness as expressed by informal collaboration.

Second, space management processes within the crowded clinic also served to reinforce power hierarchies, with oncologists claiming and being granted authority over noise level, positioning of a door, and use of desk space. Two oncologists not associated with the team regularly demanded that everyone (including team members) be quieter so they could hear better, which nonphysician team members reported finding annoying and offensive. Nonphysician clinic staff complied with (at least temporarily), but never made, such demands. This is in keeping with findings that those with higher status are more likely to issue commands and assert control over interactions (Borisoff & Merrill, 1992). The oncologist/director of the geriatric team reported that, because of his status as an oncologist, he disregarded such orders. Two oncologists (not members of the IOPOA) also occasionally asked others, in tones that implied more demanding than requesting, to vacate chairs they wished to use, but oncologists were never asked by others to move. The social worker, pharmacist, dietitian, and registered nurses asked each other for estimated duration of their work on the computers they all shared, but did not ask others to vacate the equipment. Administrative assistants expressed willingness to surrender equipment and space to all other clinic personnel (except nursing assistants, who did not use phones, computers, or desk space) with comments such as, "I'll be done in just a minute" or "I'll get out of your way" before being asked to move. As a person of provisional status in the clinic, I vacated a chair anytime I saw clinic personnel looking for a place to sit; I was willingly complicit to preserve my access to the clinic. This pecking order of privilege was carefully maintained throughout my period of observation.

Next, all team information was funneled toward the oncologists, reinforcing their higher status and problematizing the nurse practitioner's. Although other team members made interventions for patients (e.g., changing timing of medication), the oncologists made decisions regarding oncology treatment. Oncologists had no duty to report their findings to other team members before implementing a plan, but all other team members were required (directly [nurse practitioner] or indirectly [others]) to report information to the oncologist. This pattern of formal reporting (although generally effective in facilitating patient care) enhanced the oncologists' authority and privilege relative to the other team members. The two team oncologists could solicit input and include others in decision-making; however, the decision making power was theirs alone to determine how much or little input to seek. Researchers note that, although information is gathered from and direct assistance given to patients by multiple team members, the information and assessments gathered and formulated by other professionals are also part of and integral to the physician–patient interaction and affects satisfaction of both physician and patient (McCormick et al., 1996; Miller, Morley, Rubenstein, Pietruszka, & Strome, 1990). Physicians depend on the data and opinions of the other team members in making treatment decisions; the reverse is not true to the same degree.

Finally, team members reinforced physician privilege through their explanation of the IOPOA program to patients and patients' companions. Although nonphysician team members introduced themselves to patients by first name, often without also offering their last names, physicians were always referred to using the formal title of doctor with her or his last name by team members talking with patients and patients' companions (and by the physicians). Of course this pattern of naming is not unique to the IOPOA, but pervades health care systems; nurses are not addressed using a title, and it is rare for physicians to offer patients the opportunity to address them by their first names. Status differences also were reinforced through explanations of the team nature of the initial office visits, particularly with patients and/or companions who were resistant to seeing the entire team. Nonphysician team members, often the registered nurse, or whomever happened to enter the patient's room first, explained the importance of the comprehensive geriatric assessment provided by the team by saying that the process is "necessary for helping the physician to develop the most effective treatment plan." This strategy, although often effective at gaining patient compliance with the team structure for the appointment, framed all the other team members as data gatherers for the physicians instead of health care providers who provided important screenings, information, and services. In this way, team members linguistically fostered a sense that everything leads up to the climax of the physician's visit.

When a team performance upholds official values, in this case, of Western medical system's primacy of physician power, Goffman (1959) suggested it can be seen as a ceremony that reaffirms the values of the community. This ongoing ceremony, as played out in the IOPOA team, socially constructs and reaffirms the value of the physician. The need to question the continued privileging of the physician role over other disciplines is crucial for research, theorizing, and practice of health communication. Despite the dynamic negotiation of communication in the backstage, some traditional values of the Western medical establishment continue to be reinscribed through talk by the team members. Even with deliberate efforts by both IOPOA oncologists to respectfully collaborate with other team members in decision making, status differences continue to problematically place physicians in the most powerful positions. Physicians on the IOPOA team, particularly the oncologist who directs the program, have more power to assert their will in collaboration than do other team members (again despite their efforts to be egalitarian). Physicians can and do overrule other team members in decision making for patients' treatment plans. Team members appeared quite comfortable in taking orders from the physicians, but did not give orders to the physicians. The physicians also earn significantly more than the other team members. Certainly some would argue that this income and power disparity is appropriate because of the length and cost of medical education and the legal and ethical liability that physicians bear. Whether one agrees that the differences in prestige should or should not exist, they unarguably do exist (du Pre, 1999; Wear, 1997).

A corollary to the continued glorification of the physician is the continued devaluation of the work of members of other disciplines. Assessments and interventions by nonphysicians were treated as preliminary by patients and often dismissed through team communication.

Powerful Ambiguity: The Nurse Practitioner's Role

Although the oncologists' power was clear to all, the nurse practitioner's authority was far more ambiguous and problematic. Historically, physician power is associated with men and masculinity (although there are now many female physicians), and the vast majority of nurse practitioners are women (Allen, 1997) who are associated with a feminine ethic of care that is part of the nursing discipline's tradition and culture (Katzman, 1989; Prescott & Bowen, 1985; Stein, 1990). The position of nurse practitioner is a relatively new one, and the negotiation of control between nurse practitioners and physicians is still unresolved. Physicians tend to see nurse practitioners as physicians' helpers or extenders who should operate beneath the authority of physicians (Campbell-Heider & Pollock, 1987). This encourages continuation of the doctor–nurse game (Stein, 1967, 1990), which reinforces physician dominance, although nurses at all levels hold significant informal power and influence over diagnosis and treatment decisions (Allen, 1997; Campbell-Heider & Pollock, 1987). Recent studies demonstrate that some nurse practitioners and physicians have collaborated successfully (and cost-effectively) in providing long-term care to patients (Burl, Bonner, Rao, & Khan, 1998; Ryan, 1999) and that such collaborations may improve efficiency of patient care in primary care practices (Arcangelo, Fitzgerald, Carroll, & Plumb, 1996). However, the medical establishment hierarchy remains naturalized; the nurse practitioner's power (associated with the feminine) is rendered problematic and secondary to physicians'.

The IOPOA nurse practitioner had a great deal of control over what information was presented to the oncologist. Although the nurse practitioner did not officially have any supervisory power over other team members, her duties included responsibility for evaluating and reporting others' information and impressions. Team members appeared to have (and three articulated) an awareness of the nurse practitioner's status as immediately below the oncologists in terms of power, prestige, and responsibility. However, they did not perceive of her as being in authority over them. As literature on teamwork indicates, ambiguity about authority may cause significant tension and conflict (Campbell-Heider & Pollack, 1987; Hannay, 1980; Kulys & Davis, 1987). Team members negotiated their roles and power, particularly as established members departed and new ones joined the team. The nurse practitioner's role was the most challenging to demarcate because she exercised power over the other team members, but she lacked the authority to give orders. In daily practice, her power often was contested or resented, rather than accepted or taken for granted as the power of the oncologists was.

The most significant exercise of nurse practitioner power came through her role as the gatekeeper through which other team members report information to the oncologist. Team members sometimes sought direct communication with the oncologists regarding a particularly ill or at-risk patient, but for every patient they were required to formally report to the nurse practitioner specific pieces of information (e.g., screening test scores) and significant issues that warranted attention or could affect the treatment plan. The nurse practitioner then decided how much or how little of other team members' knowledge to pass on to the oncologist.

The nurse practitioner also used proxemics (use of space) to assert power over nonphysician team members and other clinic staff. At the start of each clinic session, the nurse practitioner typically claimed a desk space with stacks of files and films (e.g., CT scans) and sometimes personal items, such as a coffee mug. Unlike other team and clinic staff members, she did not remove her materials each time she got up to see a patient. Instead, her materials marked a spot as hers for the duration of the clinic session. This may sound like a trivial action, but it is actually a highly meaningful one. The clinic was an extremely crowded area, and negotiation of space was an ongoing daily process. As I mentioned earlier, I always had the sense of being in someone's way simply by standing or sitting in the desk area, and I regularly observed physicians attempting to move into areas they wished to use, heard (nonphysician) staff ask each other if they "could squeeze in" to a space at a counter, noticed staff frequently scanning the backstage clinic area for a spot to work in, and even noted several instances in which the team's pharmacist left the clinic briefly to work in her office (unlike the other team members, her office was in the same building as the outpatient clinic near the clinic pharmacy) because there was no room for her to compile her patient notes. To make a day-long claim for space and have it respected is a definite mark of power. At the same time, that claim is a mark of responsibility; the nurse practitioner is the team's information coordinator, and it is she who keeps track of the majority of the patients' records. Hence, needing a place for her extensive materials is due to her clinical role and responsibilities, and that role was recognized by other team members and clinic staff as deserving of spatial accommodation.

In other ways, the nurse practitioner's power was resisted or even challenged directly. Nonphysician team members did not recognize the nurse practitioner as having supervisory power over them. For instance, the first nurse practitioner I observed reported in her interview that when she disliked the manner in which a particular team member communicated with patients, she felt she had a responsibility to confront her about it. The team member was resentful and did not agree to change. The nurse practitioner did not have the authority to order her to adapt her behavior, and the two of them experienced tension off and on until (for other reasons) that nurse practitioner resigned. I observed the second nurse practitioner experience a different type of resistance to her power. In this case, the nurse practitioner's knowledge was challenged and steps were taken to correct her work without her consent. For example, the team's pharmacist claimed that she altered some chemotherapy prescriptions the nurse practitioner had written to improve their clarity for the pharmacists who prepared the chemotherapy agents. The nurse practitioner discovered this when she saw the altered prescriptions and inquired as to why they had been changed. The pharmacist took it on herself to review and edit chemotherapy prescriptions periodically, without first informing the nurse practitioner; in contrast, the pharmacist did not review or change physicians' orders. Clearly, the pharmacist did not perceive the nurse practitioner's authority or power to be equal to the physicians'.

The ambiguity surrounding the nurse practitioner's level of authority made it difficult for team members to communicate effectively; at the same time, the oncologists' unquestioned power constrained communication opportunities. In both cases, open discussion of power, responsibility, and decision-making authority would benefit team members.

Power, Conflict, and Team Members' Communication Style

Team members' communication with each other within the backstage largely reflected characteristics that gender scholars such as Tannen (1990) and Wood (2005) identified with feminine modes of communication. Feminine communication styles reflect values and practices traditionally associated with women, and they continue to be more prevalent among women. However, gendered styles are not dictated by biology and can be adopted by either sex. Feminine speech characteristics include expressions of equality; showing support for others; attention to the relationship level of communication; conversational maintenance work (active listening, facilitating conversation); inclusivity and responsiveness; a personal, concrete style; and a degree of tentativeness (Wood, 2005). For example, the nurse practitioner and pharmacist both made sure I felt welcome to participate in team lunches by urging me to accompany them into the serving line. Also the dietitians, social workers, and pharmacist expressed their views about a patient or other issues in such a way as to acknowledge that they were open to others' views. For example, team members followed statements of their impressions with "and what do you think?", inviting responses, or "but that's just what I thought," indicating an awareness that there could be more than one interpretation. All team members shared personal stories with concrete details, and all team members showed support for each other in times of personal crisis by inquiring about the status of problems, expressing hope for positive resolutions, and offering assistance if appropriate. For example, when the pharmacist's mother was experiencing mental illness, the other team members asked her about her mother's condition, expressed sympathy to the pharmacist about her emotional pain regarding the mental illness, and an oncologist offered to help by examining the mother.

Team members' backstage talk conformed to these norms, and shared expectations facilitated their communication by making communication patterns relatively predictable. A team that used more diverse communication styles in the clinic (regardless of whether they had diverse cultural identities) might experience considerably more misunderstandings. As Wood (2005) pointed out, however, feminine norms for communication construct a norm of politeness that makes direct conflict difficult to manage. Handling disagreement can be uncomfortable because it threatens a sense of connection and can lead to a perception of lack of support for others, lack of inclusivity, and unwarranted appeals to authority. This dynamic was not unique to the team I studied. Opie (2000) reported that within one of the health care teams she observed, an

> ethos about "support" acted to considerably constrain a key professional activity [questioning other team members about their work with patients] affecting professional accountability to the team and the team's ability to engage more fully with its members' individual and collective knowledge about a client. (p. 129)

Direct confrontations between team members were rare; I witnessed only one brief incident. This reluctance to engage in direct conflict made the negative talk about the cancer center administrators stand out as a way to express frustration safely. As discussed under the troubles talk section of the relationship-building process, administrators scheduled oncologists to conduct inpatient rounds at times that interfered with their outpatient clinics, leading to rushing and scheduling difficulties for the other team members.

Thus, complaining about the administrator who put the oncologist on rounds suggested an attack on the system or a conflict with an absent party (the administrator), rather than a conflict with the oncologist who was part of the team. Other team members could then offer support for a team member's feeling of frustration over the rushed schedule without being perceived as engaging in or promoting conflict within the team. Also minor rudeness (e.g., a team member using an impatient tone when responding to a question posed by another team member) could be attributed to the near-constant rushing rather than being perceived as personal affronts. Team members did not respond with hostility or express offense when encountering mild rudeness, willing to excuse such behavior when it could be attributed to time pressure. The crowded space and hectic pace of the clinic was not conducive to careful negotiation of disagreements, and team members avoided open conflict as the easiest, most efficient way to handle disagreements. Also, team members' avoidance of conflict did not permit public dissent that "embarrasses the reality sponsored by the team" (Goffman, 1959, p. 86). Although the primary audience for the team's performance are the patients and companions, professional colleagues work alongside the team in the backstage of the clinic (e.g., other oncologists, nurses). Goffman pointed out that all backstage regions are in a sense the frontstage for other performances, and the other cancer center personnel constituted an audience for the team as they communicated in the backstage.

Providers, Patients, and Power

Enactment of power was not confined to communication among team members and other clinic staff. A problematic effect of backstage teamwork is its powerful manifestations in frontstage communication with patients and their companions. In addition to its potential for improving patient care, backstage communication also increases health care providers' power over patients, undermining patient autonomy. In chapter 3, I detailed three specific ways in which backstage communication affects frontstage communication: (a) Team members develop beliefs and attitudes about patients before they meet them, (b) team members modify their agenda for their visit with a patient, and (c) team members receive assistance with practical facilitation of communication with patients. In this section, I explore how these relationships between backstage and frontstage relate to power.

As with the issues of power within team communication, I am not suggesting that the fact that these processes reflect systems of power and privilege means that teams should abandon them or even discount the beneficial effects of these uses of power. I am suggesting that the use of power is not irrelevant, and that awareness of power dynamics should be one of many critical factors that team members reflect on as they conduct assessments and provide care. Rather than criticizing anyone for having (or not having) certain types or expressions of power, the goal is for health care providers to be aware of and make conscious decisions about when and how to express, resist, share, and/or cede power in communication with patients and companions.

The paternalism–autonomy dialectic in the health care provider–patient relationship is certainly not unique to team interventions (e.g., Waitzkin, 1984). Structurally, all health care providers have power over patients, in that they occupy a position of expertise vis-á-vis patients who need that expertise. Although effective physician–patient communication is critical to quality health care (Ellingson & Buzzanell, 1999; Mann, 1998; Wyatt, 1991), traditionally there is an asymmetrical relationship that places the physician in authority while the patient is passive—a power dynamic that is exacerbated further when the physician holds more social status because of gender, class, race/ethnic, or age differences (Borges & Waitzkin, 1995; du Pre, 1999; Fisher, 1986; Kreps & Thornton, 1992) and is always a potential problem for older patients, toward whom physicians may exhibit ageist attitudes and behavior (Beisecker, 1996; Hummert & Nussbaum, 2001).

The interdisciplinary team–patient relationship differs from the dyadic physician–older patient relationship both positively and negatively. Team care may provide more autonomy for patients and a less intense one-on-one relationship, which some older people seem to prefer (Siegel, 1994). With a team, patients are able to direct concerns to staff members with whom they are more comfortable, and they may feel less dependent on a single health care provider. However, patients may feel uncertainty about which team member to contact for a particular issue, repetition of history and multiple visits may be necessary, and patients may give conflicting information to different team members, causing confusion (Siegel, 1994).

Although improving patient care was the goal of embedded teamwork in the clinic (as accomplished through backstage communication among team members), such teamwork nonetheless increased the power that team members had over patients in their roles as health care providers. I describe four specific ways in which their power was increased.

First, power is exercised over the patients when providers communicate with them from a position of knowledge and expertise that is exacerbated by the (beneficial) sharing of information and impressions by team members in the backstage. Health care providers exercise power over patients by virtue of their expert knowledge that the patients need. Sharing of information and impressions in the backstage increases the body of knowledge that team members work from and further enhances the expert authority that the team members had. For example, the registered dietician's knowledge of diabetes was supplemented through interaction with the clinical pharmacist concerning insulin and other diabetes medication.

Second, backstage communication and teamwork provided team members with prior warning of patients' personality and affect. This afforded team members time to plan how to communicate and be prepared to handle difficult situations. Team members knew what to expect when they entered a room and were not often caught by surprise. In contrast, patients (and their companions), waited and then coped with whomever happened to walk through their examination room door. Although I observed team members greeting and interacting with patients politely, even when faced with reluctance, rudeness, or outright hostility, team members did have varying communication styles and different tasks that they needed to accomplish with patients through communication. Patients and companions had to adjust to communication styles in the midst of the interaction, whereas team members often had time to prepare so that they could accommodate the expected style based on reports from team members.

Next, team members exerted power over patients through proxemics and space; team members could come and go as they wished, but patients were tightly controlled and kept in their rooms; they did not have freedom of movement. This restriction was exacerbated by backstage communication because the team regrouped to communicate, and the patients could not check their thoughts and reactions with others, could not take a break, and could not control the flow of people in and out of their examination room; they were subject to the comings and goings of others. Often the comprehensive geriatric assessment process was extremely time-consuming, and the patients had no input into the process.

Finally, and to me most troubling, team member power was increased by the opportunity to advance an agenda of persuasion by reinforcing ideas among team members (requesting reinforcement of a message). Team members strategized (often extensively) out of patients' presence about how to persuade patients to adopt or discontinue specific behaviors. The persuasive power wielded by team members is problematic because it gives team members further rhetorical advantage over patients who already face status and knowledge differences that privilege medical professionals in their interactions (Adelman, Greene, Charon, & Friedmann, 1992). The IOPOA team members requested reinforcement of messages to certain patients because they wanted to help the patients to be healthy; that is, their goal in the use of this power was an altruistic one. Still such strategic communication intentionally marginalizes the patients (and their companions) by excluding them from the conversation.

Yet patients were not completely powerless. At the same time that team members were exercising power over patients, the patients responded to it through resistance, compliance, or a mixture of both. They made choices, refused treatments, expressed diverging views, and otherwise resisted team members' power. Additionally, because the IOPOA team worked in an outpatient setting, recommendations were made to patients who then had time to consider options before they made decisions, enhancing their autonomy.

Patients and their companions also largely complied with and reinforced the disciplinary hierarchy among team members. Some patients and companions appeared to view the interactions with nonphysician health care professionals as relatively unimportant preambles to the physician visit (Ellingson, 2002). Consequently, they remained uninvolved in interactions with nonphysician team members unless directly asked a question. One adult son who accompanied his mother read business reports and a newspaper throughout his mother's interactions with team members, putting his reading aside and introducing himself only when the physician came into the room. On other occasions, companions actually physically left the examination room to stretch their legs or get something to eat, intending to return when the physician arrived. Companions who physically or psychologically disengaged with the nonphysician team members may have perceived that, because the other team members could not answer treatment questions or provide certain types of information, the information and interventions they did provide was of little use. People in the United States are still socialized to think of physicians as powerful authority figures (Brody, 1992), and the other team members may have seemed to play preliminary or insignificant roles compared with the physician. Some patients and companions thus appeared to grant the other team members less legitimacy and simply declined to pay attention to them. I frequently heard patients and their companions ask nonphysician team members when the doctor would be coming.

Other patients and companions reacted in the opposite manner, becoming less animated, contributing less to the conversation, and asking fewer questions when the physician was present than when the other team members were present. This may be another manifestation of socialization not to question the authority of physicians or take up "too much" of their time. Physician presence may have caused patients and companions to become more attentive to the interaction, and yet be less willing to engage in more active roles. The reluctance to be an advocate, or pursue a specific agenda, did not appear to be a result of complete understanding or satisfaction with information presented by the physician. To the contrary, after the physician left, patients and companions not infrequently turned to me and asked me to repeat information or provide further explanation.[7]

I do not believe that the pattern of deference to the authority of the physician generally reflected a lack of respect for the nonphysician team members. Many patients and companions appeared to enjoy the comprehensive interdisciplinary assessment process, and they often thanked the various professionals for talking with them, answering questions, and taking psychosocial concerns seriously. Rather, the respect for the nonphysicians was not accompanied by the same level of intimidation or respect for authority as these patients and companions may have experienced with the physicians.

---

[7]Of course it would be inappropriate for me to provide explanations or opinions. I always offered to get the registered nurse or nurse practitioner to answer their questions.

The marginalization of patients and family members' perspective within team meetings has been highly criticized by some scholars of teamwork (Opie, 1998). A similar criticism could be made of backstage teamwork, which fosters repetition and modification of messages designed to move patients toward a particular decision, gives team members time to adjust expectations that is denied to patients, and generally enhances team members' power over their patients. Clearly, although backstage teamwork enhances team members' effectiveness, the ethical dimensions of it warrant future research and reflection.

POWER AND CRYSTALLIZATION: MULTI-METHOD/MULTI-GENRE HEALTH CARE RESEARCH

Now that I have discussed how power was manifested in the backstage and frontstage of the IOPOA clinic, I want to turn the lens of power on myself and my research process. Each methodology comes with its own constraints, opportunities, epistemologies, and aesthetics. Indeed in qualitative analysis and writing, " . . . each practice makes the world visible in a different way" (Denzin & Lincoln, 2000, p. 4). Juxtaposing different conceptualizations of the same topic has sparked my imagination and articulated concepts and relationships. I have formed complex and "thoroughly partial" (Richardson, 2000) understandings of team communication as it is practiced in the backstage of the clinic and of the relationship between backstage and frontstage communication in the clinic. The richness of my approach has enabled me to articulate specific implications for interdisciplinary health care team collaboration and for writing qualitative research.

As I tacked among topics and genres, developing and writing my findings, it became increasingly apparent that both the content and form(s) of my text reproduced (even as they resisted) existing power structures within the academy and the U.S. medical system. All texts do this in some way, of course. Each genre privileges one or more epistemologies and ontologies (e.g., Denzin, 1997; Richardson, 2000). In the same way, each of my knowledge claims reflects specific "situated knowledges"—that is, perceptions of the world from an individual's particular standpoint (Haraway, 1988).

Through crystallization, I indulge in temporarily forgetting (Ferguson, 1993) the conventions of establishing truth in each genre (e.g., an evocative and coherent story; well-articulated and supported analysis). The presence of multiple genres, and the contrasts and overlap between them, point to the lack of a single objective truth. The existence of each form and its criteria for knowledge production implicates the other forms as not objective—as not the only way to represent findings. Themes or processes (grounded theory) reflect the presence of specific incidents in the data on which generalizations are formed; incidents selected for telling as stories imply larger social issues and systems of sense-making in the details of the story. The contrasts among genres make evident their mutual dependence for definition; put simply, we cannot have good without evil—without one, the other is incomprehensible. Likewise, personal, openly subjective accounts are recognized as subjective *because* more detached accounts exist. My body is silent in the grounded theory analysis *because* it is present in the narrative ethnography, *because* it is highlighted as intricately involved in my production of knowledge about teamwork in the autoethnography, and so on. Describing the multiple genres of this text as mutually productive, mutually dependent constructions that are equally useful and yet equally partial troubles the rigid methodological hierarchy of hard research over soft and scientific over interpretive. In doing so, I resist the power of experts who maintain dichotomous views of research methods. At the same time, I am complicit with other systems of power; my position as author of this book is not innocent or in some way removed from the politics of power (Haraway, 1988). *All* research and writing reflects a "will to power over truth" (Foucault, 1977/1996) or the authority to enforce one's version of reality as the authoritative one. In resisting traditional categories, I engage in resistance to power (itself a form of power) and claim the power to name an alternative approach—a truth of juxtaposing and deconstructing generic boundaries to simultaneously problematize and celebrate them as "thoroughly partial."

Through my strategy of crystallization, a much broader view of health communication is possible than if scholars strictly keep our illness narratives out of our literature reviews and our statistics away from our stories. Miller and Crabtree (2000) called for qualitative and quantitative studies in medicine and health care to form a double helix in which they are intertwined, conducted jointly to address the same or similar issues, and then used reflexively to interpret, contextualize, and problematize each other. I extend their argument by resisting the dichotomy and essentializing of quantitative and qualitative research. Instead I promote not just a double helix, but a many-faceted crystal that acknowledges that all methods and genres are constructed and inescapably privilege modes of power. In refusing to subscribe to a single mode of truth, I disrupt the taken-for-grantedness of health communication research. Researchers in health communication need to integrate narrative knowing with analytical knowing, and in the process question our acceptance of dualistic thinking that marks these modes as dichotomous in the first place. Rejecting traditional rational analysis in favor of narratives (or the reverse) simply reifies the existing dichotomy while claiming to subvert it; it is far more radical to refuse the socially constructed opposition.

Still I certainly have not escaped the system of power in medicine even with my combination of genres. All of the narrative, analysis, and essay within this text is embedded within the medical system that it explores. Although I troubled the taken-for-grantedness of team communication by revealing socially constructed aspects of the system (Gergen, 1994), I too was (and still am) caught up in its norms and expectations. This became apparent as I composed my different accounts and realized that all of them—despite their different genres and epistemologies—presented the world of the IOPOA in ways that are still well within the frame of the medical establishment. Whether I wrote stories, analysis, or personal reflection, I left unquestioned far more than I was able to problematize. Even having participated in health care settings from both patient and researcher perspectives, I still have difficulty thinking outside the box and not assuming the norms of the clinic. This immersion in the system's truths is neither incidental nor the result of a distinctly personal failure. It is impossible for anyone, no matter how reflexive, to completely escape her or his standpoint. At the same time, acknowledgment of the ways in which power operates to promote certain perspectives and silence others is vital to the construction of an ethnography.

I participated in the perpetuation of physician power too in my fieldwork and in this text. I followed the lead of those around me, addressing the physicians by their titles and last names and the other team members by their first names; in the narrative ethnographic and autoethnographic accounts, I followed this same convention. In writing analysis, I grouped all team members except the oncologists together under the label *nonphysicians* as shorthand, obscuring the distinctions between their disciplinary roles and reifying (through language) an artificial dichotomy between physician (powerful) and nonphysician (less powerful). I identified more with (and was less intimidated by) the younger female team members and therefore spent more of my time talking with them in the backstage. As was evident in the encounter with Dr. Munson related in chapter 2, I respected (and feared) the authority of physicians in the clinic and submitted to their control over the backstage along with the other less powerful personnel.

My complicity was due in part to the laudable (or at least understandable) goal of wanting to retain access to my ethnography site (Coffey, 1999). Attempts to subvert clinic norms would not have been welcomed. Although I might have caused people to stop and think, breaking unstated rules likely also would have caused me to be perceived as a nuisance to professionals performing demanding roles at a rapid pace. My energetic debate over religion and gender with Dr. Armani, for example, angered another physician, and I was criticized sharply by a physician on more than one occasion for the volume of my voice when speaking with other team members. Incidents such as these made me take seriously the risk of being denied continued access to the clinic. Also (the occasional playful debate with Dr. Armani aside), I generally attuned to several aspects of feminine styles of communication (Tannen, 1990; Wood, 2005) in my communication with team members—showing support for others, performing conversational maintenance work (active listening and facilitating the flow of conversation), paying attention to the relational level of communication, and demonstrating inclusivity and responsiveness to others—that were far more conducive to upholding social norms than to challenging them.

My presence in the clinic potentially was subversive; a researcher of communication calls attention to everyday communication and assumptions (Frey, 1994). Moreover, some aspects of this book challenge norms of the clinic by shedding light on implicit and unstated norms and practices (Gergen, 1994; Putnam, 1994). Ultimately, my complicity with power probably outweighs my revolutionary potential, but I have hope that my feminist insights and stories might be one of the multiple beginnings that work together to produce significant change within the medical establishment (Foucault, 1977/1996).

CONCLUSION

In conclusion, this chapter addressed the opportunities and limitations of the current organization and ideology of the medical establishment as a context for interdisciplinary teamwork. I contend that limitations of teamwork documented by researchers of health care teams (e.g., Opie, 1997) are due in large part to the inability or unwillingness of health care organizations to move outside of traditional patterns of power and control when organizing and implementing teams. Disciplinary power differences, rooted in historical gender and racial hierarchies, persist and limit the effectiveness of teamwork by constraining communication. Embedded teamwork, although beneficial, reflects power dynamics both within the team and between team members and patients. Acknowledging how power manifests itself in teamwork is a critical step toward reconceptualizing possibilities for improving both patient care and the well-being of health care and social service providers. The process of researching teams is also implicated as power-laden; supposedly objective study of teamwork outcomes denies the complexity of teamwork processes. Studying embedded teamwork reveals not only that teamwork is enmeshed in power dynamics, but that the process of research—what questions are asked, how studies are designed, what claims are made on the basis of data, what form or genre findings are presented in—also reflects the power and privilege of researchers.

6

CONCLUSIONS
AND
IMPLICATIONS

Throughout this book, I have described the workings of a team as they provided comprehensive geriatric assessment to geriatric oncology patients. I have stressed the importance of attending to embedded teamwork in the clinic backstage and its implications for the frontstage of the clinic. In this concluding chapter, I explore the key theoretical and practical implications of this work for understanding and engaging in teamwork. Although my findings are specific to health care settings, the central nature of backstage communication to teamwork and the relationship between the backstage and frontstage of teamwork has implications that could be applied to any context in which team members work together (backstage) to provide a service (frontstage). First, I address the need to acknowledge embedded teamwork in both health care organizations and models of teamwork. Second, I offer some conclusions on the relationship between the frontstage and backstage of the clinic. Next, I consider the need to complement teamwork research by exploring patients' perspectives on communication among team members. Then I offer some insights from this work for the new field of feminist gerontology, and I conclude with some final thoughts.

EMBEDDED TEAMWORK

The findings presented here have important implications for the formation, training, and management of teams in health care settings. Teams should recognize the communication among team members outside of team meetings as part of the fluid process of teamwork, rather than ignoring or discounting such communication as apart from or preliminary to the real teamwork that occurs in meetings. Health care organizations formed interdisciplinary teams to address the need for coordination of information and assessment for patients with complex health management needs, such as geriatric oncology patients (e.g., Cott, 1998). However, such organizations have often not adapted related systems and structures within the organization that affect the abilities, motivation, accountability, and recognition of professionals carrying out their roles as team members (e.g., time allotments, resolving scheduling conflicts). Kreps (1980, 1990), drawing on Weick's (1969) classic model of organizing, suggests that organizations whose goals or purposes necessitate responding to complex (equivocal) information inputs must accommodate employees' need for information-processing strategies that reflect a similar degree of complexity.

Clearly, providing comprehensive care to patients necessitates a great deal more communication and information processing among subsets of team members than is provided for within the administration-sanctioned 1-hour weekly meeting. The amount of patient information and its equivocality was enormous particularly given the number of screenings and assessments contributed by the team members representing a range of disciplines. IOPOA team members addressed their information-processing needs by enacting backstage communication processes that are ignored and hence not rewarded or accommodated by cancer center administration. Indeed the administration continued to make requirements of team members that made it extremely difficult for needed communication to take place, such as requiring the oncologists to periodically perform inpatient rounds during their scheduled outpatient clinic times and requiring the clinical pharmacist to be on call to the chemotherapy infusion center pharmacy during the time she worked in the IOPOA clinic. Thus, the administration recognized that geriatric oncology care is complicated, as evidenced by the formation of the interdisciplinary team, while neglecting to fully appreciate the degree of that complexity and the communicative needs it generates among team members. Fostering interaction among those employees responsible for processing equivocal information is critical to successful organizational functioning (as evidenced in this case by good patient outcomes; Kreps, 1990).

Documenting, reporting, and discussing embedded teamwork processes both within the team and to administrators is necessary to bring about change in the organizational structures that support (or fail to support) teamwork. Recognition could include documenting dyadic or triadic interactions by briefly logging date, time, topic, and participants in a team member's daily planner or notebook; compiled periodically, these data would support team members' requests to administrators for (re)allocation of work time for teamwork. Periodically bringing such data into meetings for discussion also would enable identification of trends in topics that necessitate frequent out-of-meeting interactions—such knowledge could lead to anticipating and preventing some problems by implementing changes to meeting agendas or procedures to address recurring issues. By recognizing such fleeting, dyadic, or triadic communication among team members as impacting on team relationships and process, both team members and administrators can value and reward this professional work and strategize on how to maximize its effectiveness. Currently, the IOPOA team's embedded teamwork is not acknowledged in time allotment for team members, all but one of whom (the nurse practitioner) have duties related to other departments and/or other teams. Acknowledging teamwork outside of meetings could lead to schedule adjustments that would increase employee work satisfaction and increase team members' availability to collaborate on patient care in the clinic backstage. Ultimately, increased facilitation of embedded teamwork could result in time savings for team members as more efficient communication processes are developed for addressing information-processing needs.

Management of teams within health care organizations must accommodate the complexity of the tasks faced by teams if patients are to reap the benefits of effective teamwork and health care professionals are to maximize their work satisfaction. Accommodating embedded teamwork within the everyday practice of interdisciplinary care is a practical step toward accomplishing that goal. Recognition of embedded teamwork is also needed within the theoretical approaches to studying teamwork utilized by health care, human services, and communication professionals.

MODELS OF TEAMWORK

Stage models developed by social work, nursing, and medicine as well as the bona fide group model developed by communication scholars benefit from incorporation of the embedded teamwork concept. In addition to its heuristic value, the concept points to useful directions for future research.

Stage Models

Stages of cross-disciplinary collaboration developed by theorists such as Opie (1997; i.e., multidisciplinary, interdisciplinary, transdisciplinary) function as a useful heuristic for health care researchers and are widely cited by researchers in social work, medicine, nursing, pharmacy, dietary, rehabilitation, and mental health. However, such theories do not account fully for the dynamic nature of teamwork. Although models of interdisciplinary teamwork mention that informal communication occurs in interdisciplinary teams, there is no explication of what that would involve or how it influences the dynamism of teamwork. Teams do not attain the level of interdisciplinary, for example, and consequently work in that mode. Realistically, there will be good and bad days for teamwork, and there will be some patients for whom teamwork will be more effective than for others. Moreover, some members of a given team will be more willing than others to blur boundaries, openly negotiate roles, and learn from each other (e.g., the team pharmacist blurred disciplinary boundaries with the dietitian more often than with the social worker). Such fluctuations can be accounted for and their influence considered more fully with attention to embedded teamwork practices. Moving beyond the formal meeting expands what counts as teamwork, and hence enables teams both to work in dyads and triads when they deem such collaboration to be beneficial for patient care and to frame such communication as teamwork.

Moreover, embedded practices are more flexible than meetings for navigating the hierarchical medical system. Authors call for boundary blurring, role flexibility, and dynamic teamwork structures to improve health care teamwork by bridging the gaps that persist when team members socialized in different disciplines dismiss, devalue, or misunderstand each other's discipline-specific knowledge claims (Opie, 2000; Siegel, 1994). If the rigid divisions of health care disciplines, and the hierarchy which privileges physician knowledge and power over other disciplines (e.g., Cott, 1998; Griffiths, 1998), are ever to be renegotiated, embedded teamwork through backstage communication may be a good place to start. The fluidity of backstage settings forms contexts in that disciplinary boundaries can more easily waffle, and micronegotiations can take place without a large audience (as in a meeting). Despite considerable constraints related to the crowded and hectic environment of the backstage, backstage communication moved the team from a multidisciplinary mode (acting in parallel, keeping each other informed) toward an interdisciplinary or transdisciplinary mode where (some) professional boundaries were blurred and roles negotiated (Opie, 1997). By attending to communication within embedded teamwork practices, researchers will be better able to determine the degree and types of interdependency and boundary blurring that occurs among team members.

Bona Fide Group Model

Furthermore, acknowledging and exploring embedded teamwork extends bona fide group theory in a useful direction for communication scholars bringing our unique perspective to bear on the study of groups and teams in a myriad of settings, including health care. Lammers and Krikorian (1997) expanded on Putnam and Stohl's (1990) original model of bona fide groups by articulating implicit aspects of the model via their study of surgical teams. Lammers and Krikorian argued that studies of bona fide groups must involve attention to the group in its specific institutional context because a given team task or decision "is a manifestation of much individual, small group, organizational, and institutional work that goes on prior to and after [it]" (p. 36). To continue along that path, embedded teamwork practices—those that dyads and triads of team members carry out in the backstage of medical (or other) work—involve communication among team members that is just as much a part of the team's discourse and history as that which occurs in meetings. Such embedded practices are part of the "ongoingness" of the team (Berger & Luckmann, 1966; Lammers & Krikorian, 1997). Attention to ongoing communication among team members outside of meetings enables recognition of the embedded nature of teamwork within a context in which team members spend the vast majority of their time *not* in team meetings, but in accomplishing the work that is planned, reviewed, and evaluated in team meetings. I do not doubt the centrality of meetings to the accomplishment of teamwork through communication. However, an exclusive focus on meetings suggests an artificial demarcation between team communication in meetings and communication among team members in other backstage spaces. My study of an interdisciplinary geriatric team indicates that team members do not experience these forms of communication as separate, but as coexisting in a dynamic system. Thus, the permeable boundaries of bona fide teams should be considered to include communication between dyads and triads of team members regardless of whether that communication is ever brought into a meeting as a specific point of discussion.

My findings suggest that there is a need for continued research that focuses on real (bona fide) teams in action (Putnam, 1994; Putnam & Stohl, 1990). I have focused on one team's communication over an extended period of time and fluctuating membership. My research process has yielded valuable insights into team collaboration *outside of* team meetings—findings that would not be possible in studies utilizing "zero-history" groups. It was only through extended observation and getting to know my participants that I was able to appreciate the complexity of collaboration outside of the formal team meetings, where I had been trained to believe collaboration would be found. My findings are useful to practitioners in part because I constructed them from interactions embedded within the medical system instead of in a controlled environment. Further research should examine how the backstage is socially constructed and negotiated through different team structures, populations served, and health care settings. I suspect that backstage team interactions will be constructed differently in less elite environments than the one on which I focused. Moreover, because backstage communication in the

IOPOA developed haphazardly through necessity and opportunity, the specific characteristics of other contexts (e.g., size of clinic, patient scheduling process, public or private hospital) will impact on each team's development process differently. Not all forms of collaboration will be immediately obvious; researchers need to be conscious of their assumptions about what forms of communication matter. Future research also should continue to use a variety of qualitative and quantitative methods with bona fide groups to produce knowledge that complements the existing body of teamwork knowledge and questions its assumptions.

Finally, backstage communication relates to team members' work satisfaction. Scholars have reported positive correlations among health care team membership and various measures of employee satisfaction (e.g., Abramson & Mizrahi, 1996; Gage, 1998). Embedded teamwork is as much a site for what enhances or detracts from work satisfaction as formal team meetings. The backstage communication processes enhanced team members' ability to accomplish their assessment and treatment objectives with patients, increasing satisfaction with their work. Yet the analysis of power in chapter 5 demonstrated that the hierarchy is negotiated, but largely maintained, in embedded teamwork, which potentially would detract from employee satisfaction. Further research is needed to tease out the relationship between working as part of a team and employee satisfaction.

RESEARCHING AND THEORIZING LINKAGES BETWEEN FRONTSTAGE AND BACKSTAGE

By expanding the definition of what counts as teamwork, we can envision opportunities for enhancing theory and improving practice of health care provider–patient communication. An embedded teamwork approach blurs the boundary between the frontstage and backstage of health care delivery, and hence reveals both as performative. Goffman (1959) pointed out that all backstages are, in some sense, frontstages for other performances. As team members repeatedly crossed over the literal doorway between frontstage and backstage, the boundary between the performance for the patient/companion audience and the performance of teamwork was continually blurred. The performances became enmeshed and the exact threshold elusive. Theorizing frontstage and backstage as separate spheres obscures the vital connections between them. Goffman's (1959) dramaturgical theory emphasizes that the frontstage and backstage are adjacent, and both are integral to team performances. Even teams that conduct assessments and interventions asynchronously (not in the clinic backstage at the same time) are likely to carry out joint work in dyads and triads of team members outside of meetings via phone and brief, face-to-face interactions (Opie, 2000; Saltz, 1992).

These discourses should be considered as existing in a reflexive, integrated, dynamic relationship.

Theories and conceptualizations of health care teamwork must inhabit a crossroads of organizational, team, health care provider–patient, and health care provider–patient–companion communication to offer a sufficiently complex view of the world of clinics. The daily negotiation of teamwork creates a context in which frontstage and backstage communication are inseparable and mutually productive. Backstage practices such as reading and writing notes, discussing patients' affect, and sharing information and impressions influence subsequent interactions with patients. Because this cycle is continually repeated, each interaction contributes to the development the climate and culture of teamwork and health care delivery.

Extending the conceptualization of embedded teamwork further, I suggest that the line between the frontstage and backstage is a permeable boundary that is continually crossed—a point of ongoing negotiation rather than a fixed entity. As team members repeatedly cross over the literal doorway between the clinic frontstage and backstage, the two forms of communication keep intersecting. Embedded teamwork complicates the performance of health care provider and team member because the frontstage and backstage overlap. The point at which one performance (for the patient/companion audience) ends and the performance of team member/collaborator among professionals begins is elusive and transitory. The performances thus become enmeshed and need to be theorized in a clinical model of communication that reflects this complex relationship. Ideally, the repeated crossing of multiple boundaries among members of health care teams and between health care professionals and their patients (and patients' companions) will enhance collaboration by providing multiple sites for communication and connection.

To capture the richness of boundary negotiation between frontstage and backstage and the complexities of managing team and individual professional tasks, identities, and goals, researchers need to engage in methods that explore teamwork rather than, as most studies do, measuring its correlation with patient outcomes (Opie, 1997). Beyond simply complementing quantitative methods with qualitative strategies, this involves experimentation and pushing the boundaries of what counts as valid, practical, or useful research. Traditional health communication research has been largely quantitative and positivist (seeking to be objective) in its orientation (e.g., du Pre, 1999; Vanderford, Jenks, & Sharf, 1997). Scholars of communication in health care settings have paid scant attention to fleeting, informally structured communication that is difficult to document and record, preferring frontstage physician–patient communication interactions as the focus of the majority of research in health care settings (Atkinson, 1995). Our understanding of teamwork has been skewed by this preference for studying communication in a neat dyadic interaction:

the one-to-one medical consultation is a kind of synecdoche; that is, it stands in a part-for-whole relationship with the whole field of medical work. . . . Rather than diffuse and protracted, the cognitive and linguistic tasks of medicine are all too easily summarized as if they were virtually simultaneous events. (Atkinson, 1995, p. 35).

As researchers, we look for and recognize data as bounded, scheduled, formal communication in team meetings—the closest we can come to the dyadic physician–patient interaction—and we have separated it for research and theory building from other types of communication. Thus, our methods are well suited to meetings—we record, transcribe, and painstakingly analyze the communication in meetings. Whether quantitative or qualitative, such analysis generally focuses on identifying and coding or categorizing the norms, rules, and communicative processes used to make group decisions about an individual patient's care; the goal is to assess the quality of the decisions made. This important work is only one aspect of teamwork. To understand what team members do during all but the 1 or 2 hours per week they spend in the team meeting, researchers must cast a wider net. A broader range of methodology allows for a more complex and thorough understanding of the meanings of health care (Miller & Crabtree, 2000).

My study of the IOPOA attempted to do just that—to study as holistically as possible how one team communicated within itself *and* with its patients. Ethnographic data are openly subjective, which tends to make health care providers trained in scientific methodology uneasy. Having gone still farther away from claims of scientific objectivity by introducing narrative and personal (autoethnographic) writing strategies, I have undoubtedly pushed the envelope beyond what can easily be accepted by more traditional researchers and practitioners. I do not view different approaches to research as competing with each other, however. It is not my intention that the qualitative and interpretive analysis and writing presented in this book be seen as a criticism or indictment of those researchers operating at the other end of the research continuum. Instead I urge practitioners and researchers to avoid subscribing to the "law of the hammer" that is, to value a particular research method so much that they simply look for data (nails) to which they can apply their method (hammer) while ignoring all other phenomena not suited to their particular tool. Further, I urge us to value a wide range of methods and the insights that they offer.

One important aspect that my research did not address directly is patients and patients' companions' views of teamwork. Although I did pay close attention to and interact directly with patients, my writing focused on their interactions with team members to understand how the team members gather information, develop opinions, and share these opinions with other team members. Patients' and companions' behavior, as represented in the narratives and analysis, provided support for my claims about team members' communication and only implicitly revealed how patients and companions perceived of their experience with the IOPOA team. The patients' perspective is thus marginalized in the final product, although certainly I have been accurate and endeavored to be respectful in my representation of them and their companions, and, of course, my perspective is influenced greatly by my own identity and experiences as a patient. I am aware that this approach is not patient-centered; that is, it does not place patients' perceptions as primary sources of meaning (Vanderford et al., 1997)—a practice that has recently gained in popularity and one that I value highly (Ellingson & Buzzanell, 1999). Patients and family members are generally not considered to be part of teams and typically are excluded from discussions about care decisions in which they have a stake (Opie, 1998). Subsequent research should focus more on patients' and companions' perspectives on communication among team members and between team members and patients— not just in meetings, but within clinical settings.

FEMINIST GERONTOLOGY

Another important implication concerns the possibilities of embedded teamwork research for the burgeoning field of feminist gerontology. Gerontology has traditionally been dominated by (male) researchers with biomedical perspectives who carried out quantitative research (McCandless & Conner, 1999). The biomedical perspective of geriatric medicine has been challenged by interdisciplinary geriatric teams who use biopsychosocial orientations to patient care, reflected in the comprehensive geriatric assessment used (in some form) by virtually all geriatric programs. The majority of physicians in geriatrics are men, and researchers have conducted a large percentage of geriatrics research on the male Veterans Administration (VA) hospital population, excluding or marginalizing the experiences of women (Ray, 1999).

However, the giving and receiving of geriatric care is largely a woman-centered activity. Women make up the majority of geriatric patients (McCandless & Conner, 1999), and the vast majority of the direct-care providers are women (Wear, 1997). Feminist gerontology seeks to reclaim the experiences of older women, particularly in health care (Garner, 1999; Ray, 1996). I also would encourage feminist gerontologists to include in our agenda the reclaiming and critical examination of the experiences of the female health care providers who provide most of the care for these older women. As in the IOPOA, fields such as nursing, social work, and dietary—integral parts of comprehensive geriatric assessment teams—continue to be largely the province of women. My project demonstrates the richness of the team members' experiences in providing care. In particular, I was fascinated by team members' weaving of the personal and professional as they collaborated in the backstage of the clinic, sharing details of their lives as they exchanged information and opinions about patients. In less than 2 hours, team members' emotions often ran the gamut from sadness over a dying patient, to anger at an uncooperative companion, to frustration at not being able to have access to a computer, to happiness from exchanging social talk with a friend, to fatigue from being up with a sick child the night before, to satisfaction at a successful intervention. I often left the clinic so emotionally drained that I was unable to do anything but go home and rest. Yet the team members performed this work day in and day out. The work of professional caring can be satisfying, but it is also incredibly taxing (Sacks, 1988; Wood, 1994). Recognition of the gendered (and raced and classed) nature of geriatric health care can improve understanding and theorizing of communication within geriatric settings. Feminist gerontology offers a critical framework for reclaiming and valuing the work of health care providers that often goes unappreciated.

FINAL THOUGHTS

"A conclusion is the place where you got tired of thinking," according to Martin H. Fischer (cited on www.brainyquote.com). Although I am not tired of thinking about teamwork, I do contend that conclusions are always placed in a somewhat arbitrarily chosen point along the journey of a research project. Certainly, health care teams will continue to be of utmost importance in delivering care within health care organizations; as scholars, leaders, and members of teams, we should seek to improve communication and collaborative processes to maximize team effectiveness. I sought to present the richest and most holistic view possible of the IOPOA team and the people it serves, but I have made strategic choices about what issues to include and which to leave out. Moreover, through this research project, I have become a more compassionate person, and that is the greatest gift that research can offer. As a researcher grounded in my own ongoing experiences as a patient, I feel more for patients, their companions, the IOPOA team members, other cancer center personnel, other researchers, and myself. I find I am less interested in criticizing and more inclined to empathizing. I have been inspired by the warmth and caring exhibited daily by the IOPOA team, despite significant obstacles and constraints, and the vitality, strength, and humor many of the patients and companions maintained in the face of immense suffering. At the close of this project, I am more aware of the systemic problems in the medical system, but I am also more hopeful that significant change will eventually be made.

Appendix A

DETAILS OF
DATA COLLECTION

The study reported here began as a semester-long project during my doctoral program at the University of South Florida. I gained entry to the IOPOA through Dr. Carolyn Ellis, who had previously conducted preliminary fieldwork there in preparation for a grant proposal. Because of the good will among Dr. Ellis, the director of the IOPOA, and the nurse practitioner on the team at that time, I was welcomed warmly and encountered little, if any, resistance to my presence at meetings or in the clinic, despite the contrast between my qualitative approach and the team's more biomedical orientation to research. Because of my warm reception, I decided (with the team's permission) to continue participant observation in the IOPOA clinic and team meetings throughout my coursework and to make this a long-term research project. I briefly discuss feminist ethnographic practices and then provide details of my data collection.

FEMINIST ETHNOGRAPHIC PRACTICES

I specifically intended my ethnography to be a feminist one; I was interested in power dynamics among team members, between health care providers and patients (and patients' companions; see Ellingson, 2002, for a description of the roles of patients' companions in geriatric health care), and among cancer center personnel working within the clinic alongside the IOPOA team. Being familiar with analyses of gender in health communication (e.g., Gabbard-Alley, 1995) and feminist critiques of the medical establishment (e.g., Wear, 1997), I was also focused on the relationship between everyday clinic communication and the gender, race, class, and professional hierarchies that persist within health care settings.

Definitions of feminist ethnography vary (Lengel, 1998; Williams, 1993), but tend to have in common several factors that are descriptive of my approach to conducting ethnography in the IOPOA clinic. First, they tend to focus on the experience of women (Denzin, 1997; Lengel, 1998). Holman Jones (1998) argued that,

> Feminist ethnography, then, is the sought and written experience of women within and between cultures. . . . Feminist ethnography does not exclude men or men's experience, but it does typically feature women's experience. In addition, feminist ethnography is almost always done by women. . . . (p. 422)

Women's experiences in groups have been marginalized from the study of small-group and team research (Meyers & Brashers, 1994). The majority of group communication studies has been carried out using White male participants and has reflected masculine communication norms and values (Wood, McMahan, & Stacks, 1984; Wyatt, 1993; [notable exceptions include Goodwin, 2002; Lesch, 1994]). I addressed this lack of attention to women's experience in my fieldwork.

The IOPOA team was made up entirely of women with the exception of the program director. Hence, in studying the team, I was studying primarily women health care professionals. All of the certified nursing assistants (CNAs) and the administrative support personnel I encountered in the clinic were women. There were also some men present in the clinic and in team meetings; the oncologists who shared clinic space with the IOPOA or who consulted with the IOPOA on particular patients (e.g., the head of the psychiatry department) were men. Of course many of the program's patients and patients' companions were men as well. Although older women make up the majority of geriatric patients in this country (McCandless & Conner, 1999), the sex division was much more equally divided in the IOPOA. Because older women are more likely to be living in poverty than older men (Garner, 1999), they are less likely than men to have the resources necessary to travel to a regional center and less likely to have good quality insurance that would cover the cost of having treatment there. Nonetheless, I observed far more women over the course of my time in the clinic and meetings than I did men.

A second issue in feminist ethnography is an awareness of and active interrogation of power dynamics in the field setting. Discourses of power within the cancer center (and the larger context of Western medicine) present the White, male, able-bodied, heterosexual, socioeconomically privileged as simultaneously neutral/normative and as rightfully being in power (Haraway, 1988; Wear, 1997). For too long such norms in medicine went unnoted or unquestioned, and too often scholars continue to obscure such norms. For example, many writers label people's race only when it is something other than White, thus reinforcing the normativity of Whiteness. Systemic hierarchy is a crucial aspect of the context in which the team operates: Teams "are embedded within an organization's history, culture, and structure" (Barge & Keyton, 1994). The team both upholds and subverts elements of this hierarchy; this tension underlies the narrative ethnographic and autoethnographic accounts and is addressed more overtly in the analysis of power in chapter 5.

A third aspect of feminist ethnography is attention to positionality (identity, roles, and perspective) of myself as a researcher (Coffey, 1999; Reinharz, 1992). I have endeavored "to become answerable for what [I] learn how to see" (Haraway, 1988, p. 583), acknowledging and even celebrating my positionality and interrogating the relationship between my standpoints and the implicit and explicit claims I make in my writing while openly proclaiming the limitations of my view (Ellingson, 1998). Although not exclusive to feminist ethnographers, attention to the perspective of the researcher is vital to feminist research because it rejects claims to the "view from nowhere" (Haraway, 1988) espoused by positivist researchers. In practice, this attention to positionality involved continually reflecting on what I was writing and how what I noticed and documented reflected who I am. For example, because I am deeply ingrained with a patient's perspective, I considered my descriptions of health care provider–patient communication in my fieldnotes carefully to see how they might reflect a more sympathetic stance toward patients than toward team members. I did this not in an effort to remove bias, but to be as conscious as possible of how my unique self influences my perceptions.

Next, I feel a need for reciprocity with my participants—an important tenet of many types of feminist research (Reinharz, 1992). I offered team member participants the opportunity to review my findings and contribute their ideas, which were then used to refine later drafts of this book. My voice is certainly privileged over theirs in the final version of our work together, however. In addition to offering the opportunity to give feedback on findings, I attempted to give back to my participants in other ways. I gave a talk at their annual retreat on current research on health care provider–patient research, and I provided a safe sounding board for team members to vent feelings in the clinic. To the first nurse practitioner with the team, I provided significant assistance and encouragement as she began to explore qualitative research, and I conducted a pilot study with her that eventually became the foundation for her dissertation in medical anthropology. We provided mutual support and friendship to each other as we both progressed through our research projects. Giving participants a voice in research reports and providing them with feedback and/or other services is critical to most research on bona fide groups (Frey, 1994). Although I have doubtlessly received more from my participants than I have offered them, I am comfortable that participants have felt respected throughout this process.

Finally, feminist research seeks to make political and social change (Clough, 1994; Olesen, 2000; Stack, 1993). Along with other feminist researchers and many postmodern and humanist researchers, I reject the notion of value-free research (e.g., Bochner, 1994; Bochner & Ellis, 1996; DeVault, 1990; Ellis, 1997; Fine, 1988; Mies, 1983; Reinharz, 1992). I have a political agenda of questioning oppressive institutional structures and practices and of improving the quality of life for patients, companions, and health care providers. In addition to any change or consciousness raising that may result from reading my account(s) of the world of the IOPOA, feminist ethnography enables the research itself to be an intervention, particularly in medical contexts. "[Qualitative] research needs to risk restoring relationships to the clinical world. Clinical research can heal by transforming into praxis" (Miller & Crabtree, 2000, p. 628). *Praxis* refers to the intersection of theory and knowledge with practice. Therefore, health care providers communicating among themselves and with researchers in clinical settings have the potential to bring about transformation of communication patterns and norms in both the frontstage and backstage of the clinic.

DATA COLLECTION

I conducted participant observation during new patient clinics about once a week from September 1997 through August 1999, with the exception of June to August of 1998, when I was unavailable during scheduled clinic times due to my teaching schedule. I generally spent 3 to 5 hours at a time in the clinic. I also attended weekly staff meetings and generated field notes about those interactions from September 1997 to August 2000. These team meetings lasted approximately 1 hour and 15 minutes, and team members reported on each patient seen that week by the physicians. Team members also discussed other business, such as scheduling, research, grants, and visitors. In addition to the team members who work together in the clinic, a clinic administrator, an aging studies research fellow, the administrative assistant for the IOPOA, and I regularly attended the meetings. Each week a different pharmaceutical company representative provided a catered lunch for the team and spent a few minutes speaking about new products and/or product research. I continued to observe at these meetings each week after leaving the clinic to stay in contact with the team members until the interviewing phase of my research—through August 2000.

I generated extensive fieldnotes describing interactions among staff members and among staff, patients, and caregivers. While in the clinic, I initially kept "scratch notes" (Lindolf & Taylor, 2002) in a notebook and later on a "palmtop" computer. These notes recorded key words and phrases, pieces of dialogue, and other details in an informal short-hand format. Immediately after observing, I used my scratch notes and the memories they sparked to construct detailed, comprehensive fieldnotes of my experiences in the clinic and in meetings.

I also tape recorded nine patients throughout their initial visit with the IOPOA team. I approached patients for participation while in the waiting room, following procedures approved by the cancer center scientific review committee and USF Institutional Review Board. Participants were recorded interacting in the examination rooms with each member of the IOPOA. To supplement these patient recordings, I also recorded the staff meetings during which these patients were discussed. Nine of the clinic patient–team interactions were transcribed by a professional transcriptionist and edited for medical terminology and accuracy by myself. I used the transcripts to supplement my observations and notes.

Because of my commitment to feminist and humanist research principles (e.g., Reinharz, 1992), I felt strongly that the people with whom I had worked mostly closely should be given an opportunity to provide feedback on my findings, which would then be incorporated within the final draft. I asked each of the IOPOA team members with whom I had spent time in the clinic to participate in private, semistructured interviews. During and after conducting the interviews, I further refined my findings.

Lasting approximately 60 minutes, these loosely structured interviews were designed to elicit staff member perceptions of communication in the clinic setting vis-á-vis the descriptions I had developed. I shared with them Tables 3.1 and the data excerpt from chapter 3 (which were combined as one table at that time), in which I detail seven processes that describe the communication that goes on in the backstage areas of the clinic, and the relationship of these processes to team members' communication with patients and patients' companions. I also explained that I had presented these same ideas in narrative forms with the goal of complexifying my results by offering multiple views of their team. Six of the team members consented to an interview, wherein I asked the following questions:

1. Please examine this preliminary typology of backstage communication carefully. What are your initial reactions to it? Prompts:
    ◄ What do you agree or disagree with?
    ◄ What seems unclear to you?
    ◄ What have I left out or what would you add?

2. How do you see these communication practices as varying among different team members?
3. How do you think these communicative practices developed?
4. Why do you think you engage in these communicative practices with team members?
5. How is communicating with team members related to your discipline?
6. How do you think your communication in the backstage areas of the clinic is related to or affected by the context of the cancer center as an organization?

The team membership changed over the course of my time there. After August 1999, I stopped observing in the clinic, but continued to attend team meetings. In the meetings, I met an additional three new staff members, but I did not interview them because I had not observed them working in the clinic. Any views I presented of the team in action were necessarily obsolete by the time I wrote them down; the team context and practices continually adapted to face new opportunities and challenges. Because I had to draw a line somewhere to finish this project, I declined to engage the most recent additions to the team in this book. I do refer to other past team members with whom I worked, but who are no longer with the team. I conducted an extensive interview with the nurse practitioner who is no longer with the program, but, who was my primary contact for the first year I engaged in participant observation with the team. She was one of the founding members of the IOPOA and, as such, was a valuable source of background information on the team, as well as insights into how the team has changed over time. She and I developed a friendship outside of the IOPOA context and completed a separate research project together. Also she continued to substitute on a per diem basis for the current nurse practitioner when she was on vacation or traveling.

Appendix B

———————◆———————

ANALYSIS AND
WRITING PRACTICES

I was reluctant to interrupt the close juxtaposition of genres through which my findings are presented with an in-depth consideration of methodological issues, and instead I placed this important discussion here in an appendix. Having made my argument for the wonderful opportunities inherent in mixed-genre/multimethod texts, I want to offer a further discussion of how I conceive of narrative ethnography, grounded theory analysis, and autoethnography as individual methods. I discuss some of the opportunities and constraints of accounts generated from these methods as I explain each of them. Like my delineation of the backstage communication processes, I divide my methods for discussion even though I practiced them simultaneously because it enables close attention to each.

WRITING NARRATIVE ETHNOGRAPHY

———————◆———————

"Doing" narrative ethnography involves collecting the data, making sense of them, and then writing about them; these processes do not occur in a linear fashion, but are interwoven. There are many different perspectives on how researchers should behave when they are in the field. The term *participant observation* implies that the researcher is a participant in interactions, but also somehow apart from them, able to observe her or him self interacting with others. Early ethnographers argued that they took adequate measures to ensure that their scientific study of the natives was uncontaminated by their own presence and biases (Van Maanen, 1988). Few ethnographers now would argue that their presence was irrelevant to their findings, but a range of perspectives exist on what the desirable position or role of researchers is vis á vis their subjects or research participants. "Going native" is seen by some as a sign of failure of the researcher to maintain an appropriate critical distance from those being researched. However, native ethnographers now study their own cultures (Denzin, 1997). I assumed what Lindlof and Taylor (2002) called the *observer as participant* role in my fieldwork. I interacted continually with my research participants as I observed them interacting with others. My participants learned a great deal about me over time and were undoubtedly influenced by my presence in the clinic and at meetings. I developed relationships with my participants, and it is in those relationships that I learned about their worlds, invited them to glimpse mine, and entered theirs to some degree.

I use the term *research participants* consciously; the term *subjects* connotes a position much closer to the positivist end of the qualitative continuum than the one where I situate myself. The team members, their patients, the patients' companions, and the other cancer center staff actively participated in my research; they did not somehow go on about their business as I recorded it. My research was a dialogue among us, with different participants engaging me more actively than others at different times. It is through our mutual engagement that I generated data in the form of fieldnotes, audiorecordings, and my own memories.

The narrative ethnography in chapter 2 reflects elements of both realist and impressionist ethnographies (Van Maanen, 1988). Writing narrative ethnography is a process of constructing narratives from fieldnotes, memories, and other written accounts. I constructed narratives to make sense out of what I experienced. I endeavored to stay close to details of interactions as I had recorded them in my fieldnotes and in my memory. While trying to include each of the team members in at least one interaction and to give a feeling of the relationship between the backstage and frontstage, I chose stories that impressed me as interesting, meaningful, or demonstrating either the everyday mundane world of the IOPOA or the atypical but critical events that shape how the team worked together.

After discarding several other plots, I chose the frame of a "day in the life" around which to arrange the set of stories I wished to share because it enabled me to show a broader range of incidents than typically happened in a single day. I took real events and put them into a new time frame, acknowledging the partial decontextualization of the interactions and recontextualization of them into different times and in differing juxtapositions. This is an improvement over telling the story of a real day because readers get to experience a wider variety of interactions. It also works significantly better than simply stringing together a series of events on different days because the reader gets a sense of the rhythm of a day in the clinic as it is simulated in the narrative.

I openly claim that this is not a real day, but a realistic day. My goal is to have readers experience the clinic. However, I presented a collection of incidents that reflect as closely as possible actual events as I recorded and remember them. In composing this story, I chose to position myself in the story primarily as observer rather than active participant so as to keep the focus on the IOPOA team, patients, patients' companions, and other clinic staff. I sought to faithfully portray the team members in the ways that I have come to know them.

Narrative ethnographic representations of research offer readers the opportunity to see the IOPOA clinic—to get a sense of what it feels like to be there. Stories are more open than analysis; they allow readers to empathize and connect with the truths presented in the stories. Scholars such as Bochner (1994), Frank (1995), and Denzin (1997) have suggested that readers of narrative have the opportunity to read *with* a story to consider its ethical, moral, and personal implications for themselves. This mode of understanding contrasts sharply with social science writing, which does not offer readers stories, but analyses of stories. In most social science, stories are raw data to be broken apart and analyzed for generalizable truths, themes, or patterns. Narrative knowing offers more openings for readers to interpret multiple meanings from multiple positions (Bochner, 1994; Frank, 1995) and to ". . . show what it means to live in a world mediated by the contingencies of using language and fashioning an identity . . ." (Bochner, 1994, p. 21). A narrative text acknowledges and welcomes readers to generate different meanings for the text depending on their personal experiences and perspectives; readers become participants in the meaning-making (Denzin, 1997). Feminist researcher Laurel Richardson (1990) eloquently articulated the possibilities of narrative for the social sciences:

> Narrative gives room for the expression of our individual and shared fates, our personal and communal worlds. Narrative permits the individual, the society, or the group to explain its experiences of temporality because narrative attends to and grows out of temporality. It is the universal way in which humans accommodate to finitude. Narrative is the best way to understand human experience and hence the least falsifying of that experience. (p. 218)

The power of stories to communicate the human condition in an accessible, inspirational, and therapeutic way is the biggest strength of narratives.

However, using narrative ethnography to "report" research findings does not totally avoid the representational quagmire. The arrangement of fieldnotes into stories involves just as much sense-making as writing an analytic account. Indeed even the writing of fieldnotes begins the process of analysis (Wolf, 1992). Literary narratives are just as much constructions of the researcher as are academic narratives; experimental texts do not escape their authorship (Haraway, 1988). Meanings are created and inscribed through the construction of stories that impose order on unordered events (Bochner, 1994). The constraints of the genre are present when an intelligible narrative is constructed. Although stories are more open and invite more directly for the reader to fashion personal, multiple meanings, the author's positionality still underlies what is included and excluded. Representation of others is still accomplished via the author's power even if that power is altered and/or somewhat diminished through inclusion of large portions of participants transcribed words or as stories fashioned out of dialogue with participants (e.g., Fox, 1996).

> Whereas experimenting with strategies of representation has produced some alternatives, it is doubtful that these forms of representation are distinctly different from others, since the end product does not necessarily appropriate less and does not shift the balance of power or the benefits. Despite important efforts to experiment with strategies of representation and authorship, the basic power differences and distribution of benefits remain the same. (Wolf, 1992, p. 34)

I am keenly aware when I write narratives of the details I include, those I leave out, and the consequences of those decisions; I have less control over readers' interpretation of my narrative than I do over their interpretation of my analysis, but the amount of control I have is still vast. Thus ethnographic narratives offer the possibilities of evoking readers' emotions and imaginations, but still reflect authorial power.

CONSTRUCTIVIST GROUNDED THEORY

I conducted a grounded theory analysis of the set of data described in detail above. This includes fieldnotes, transcripts, dictations, and interview notes based upon my participant observation with the IOPOA from September 1997 through August 2000. In this section, I will describe in detail what I mean by *grounded theory analysis*, explain the meanings I ascribe to the analysis, and detail the processes of data analysis.

Charmaz (1990, 2000) argued persuasively that grounded theory methodology can be used in highly positivist studies, interpretive studies, or in studies positioned somewhere between those two ends of the qualitative continuum. Glaser and Strauss (1967) first described the method that was imbued with positivist assumptions of objective science that discovered existing realities through a neutral observer. In their (laudable) efforts to legitimate qualitative research, they drew on the language of quantitative sciences that emphasized objectivity, generalizability, and discovery (not construction) of truth. Both researchers revised their positions over time (Glaser, 1992; Strauss & Corbin, 1990, 1998), but both remained within positivist or postpositivist frameworks that did not incorporate postmodern, constructivist, feminist, or critical race theory critiques about the politics of the production of knowledge (Charmaz, 2000).

Charmaz (2000) summarized the critiques of grounded theory as consisting of four primary criticisms:

> . . . grounded theory method (a) limits entry into subjects' world, and thus reduces understanding of their experience; (b) curtails representation of both the social world and subjective experience; (c) relies upon the viewer's authority as expert observer; and (d) posits a set of objectivist procedures on which the analysis rests. (p. 521)

These criticisms are valid in relation to most traditional grounded theory analyses, which made explicit claims to objective truth. However, some recent work, notably Charmaz' research with people living with chronic illnesses, has eschewed the positivist framework and focused instead on the meanings created by participants and researchers. Strauss and Corbin's (1998) moved from Glaser and Strauss' strictly positivist framework to embrace some postpositivist concerns, such as including participants' voice in published accounts, striving to accurately represent participants, and recognizing the art as well as the science of analysis further by recasting grounded theory in a constructivist frame.

Charmaz (2000) went further and embraced arguments by feminist theorists and others that the positionality of the researcher is central to the construction (not discovery) of knowledge. She described a constructivist grounded theory as a method that

> recognizes the interactive nature of both data collection and analysis, resolves recent criticisms of the method, . . . reconciles positivist assumptions and postmodernist critiques . . . fosters development of qualitative traditions through the study of experience from the standpoint of those who live it . . . recognizes that the categories, concepts, and theoretical level of an analysis emerge from the researcher's interactions within the field and questions about the data . . . fosters our self-consciousness about what we attribute to our subjects and how, when, and why researchers portray these definitions as real . . . [and] sensitizes [researchers] to multiple realities and the multiple viewpoints within them. . . . (pp. 522–523)

This revised method fits within the feminist framework for my research. Such a framework allows for grounded theory methods to be adapted for interpretive studies in which the researcher openly engages her positionality and the joint construction of meaning.

Although many aspects of my positionality affect this analysis, my ideological stance as a feminist ethnographer and my perspective as a cancer survivor are particularly relevant in considering the claims I make in the text. Much of what I and other feminists object to about positivist science comes from researchers' claims of "the view from nowhere"—their all-knowing, infallible, uncontaminated Truth (Haraway, 1988). In refusing to claim discovery of Truth, I do not give up all claims to having some important ideas and thoughts to share; by being forthcoming about the *groundedness* of my grounded theory in the world I co-construct, I support my claims. In the grounded theory analysis, I moved from narrative writing into an analytical style, but I did not abandon my commitment to self-scrutiny and careful exploration of the relationship between where I see from and what I see. I next discuss how these broad goals translated into specific practices as I analyzed my data.

Charmaz (2000) explained that researchers can "form a revised, more open-ended practice of grounded theory that stresses its emergent, constructivist elements. We can use grounded theory methods as flexible, heuristic strategies rather than as formulaic procedures" (p. 510). I followed the same basic steps of traditional grounded theory research outlined by Strauss and Corbin (1990) and Charmaz (2000): coding data, developing inductive categories, continually revising the categories, writing memos to explore preliminary ideas, continually comparing parts of the data to other parts and to the related literature, collecting more data and fitting it into the categories and noting where it does not fit, and revising the categories (theoretical sampling).

I analyzed my data inductively (throughout the participant observation process), identifying emergent themes and patterns in the data. My loose categorization scheme was continually revised as I continued to read through and reflect on the data, organizing and reorganizing codes into larger categories and breaking down general categories into more specific subgroups. Although the findings in this chapter strive more to be representative of my overall understanding of the IOPOA than the narrative account, I also considered atypical events to support, problematize, and contextualize patterns in my efforts to remain aware of the process of constructing knowledge.

Analysis continued through my writing of reflections, called *memos* in grounded theory, that considered patterns and revised them. Revision continued as I began to write early drafts of my findings. As Richardson (2000) pointed out, writing is a method of inquiry, not a "mopping up" activity undertaken after the research is completed. Sense-making continued throughout the process of writing and revision. As I wrote, my ideas changed, and new insights emerged and were integrated. In addition, I incorporated participants' responses and suggestions into the final schema.

There are several advantages to this form of grounded theory method. First, it provides useful generalizations about communication processes that contribute to the body of knowledge about team communication and may prove helpful for other health care teams as they seek to revise and improve their modes of practice. This genre also allows for a relatively efficient presentation of information based on a large corpus of data; grounded theory provides a means for summarizing the experiences of a large number of people over an extended period of time. Next, the language and style of grounded theory pushes the boundaries of the positivist biomedical orientation that dominates medicine and medical research to incorporate qualitative findings. At the same time, this genre uses language that fits fairly well within the norms of medicine, helping to make the findings intelligible and more palatable, and easing scientific readers into consideration of qualitative perspectives, rather than plunging them into a radically different mode of data representation (e.g., poems or narratives). Finally, the grounded theory genre allows me to articulate arguments, to make claims and support them with data and connections to relevant literature.[1] As Wolf (1992) argued, "I still see my ethnographic responsibility as including an effort to make sense out of what I saw, was told, or read—first for myself and then for my readers" (p. 5). Grounded theory offers one useful form of sense-making that appeals to my desire for analysis.

Grounded theory (even if conceived of as constructivist) has its share of limitations of course. Traditional social science methods such as this one privilege theory over stories, reason over emotions, and the universal and distant over the specific and personal (Bochner, 1994). Denzin (1997) argued against the use of analytical methods (such as grounded theory and narrative analysis) because:

> These methods of analysis risk reproducing the fallacy of objective reading. . . . This framework presumes a fixed text with fixed meanings. . . . These methods fail to address language's radical indeterminacy, the slipperiness of signs and signifiers . . . and the fact that language creates rather than mirrors reality. . . . These methods fail to examine the text as a meaningful whole. (p. 244)

---

[1]Using grounded theory does not mean that participants' emotions are individuality are completely obscured, however. Charmaz's constructivist approach to grounded theory proproses that this method is midway between postpositivist and postmodern research methods, using postmodern theory to inform study of experience. Such research looks for "views and values as well as for acts and facts . . . beliefs and ideologies as well as situations and structures" (Charmaz, 2000, p. 525).

This privileging of the analytical ear is unacceptable to Denzin. As is apparent in my choice to include grounded theory analysis in this text, I disagree that such genres are necessarily unacceptable from an interpretive perspective. I hear in this statement echoes of critics of narrative research who assert that unscientific, personal, messy writing "must be avoided." As Bochner (1997) put it, "We know we're onto something, when we're told, 'You mustn't think that way'" (p. 425). No genre should be declared off limits; a plurality of genres can only strengthen the social sciences. However, I acknowledge the strength of Denzin's and others' position on the limitations of analytical qualitative methods; if left unexamined, unproblematized, and not complemented by other genres, detached and analytical writing offers only limited entry into understanding researchers' and participants' worlds and sense-making processes.[2] Analytic knowing must *not* be the only form of approved knowing in the social sciences, but neither should narrative knowing or any other single epistemology.

AUTOETHNOGRAPHY

The third method invoked in my exploration of the IOPOA is autoethnography (Ellis, 1997). Ellis and Bochner (2000) described autoethnography as

> an autobiographical genre of writing and research that displays multiple layers of consciousness, connecting the personal to the cultural . . . [autoethnographers focus] outward on social and cultural aspects of their personal experience; then, they look inward, exposing a vulnerable self

---

[2]Denzin acknowledged that texts are not solely constructed by authors, but are a co-construction between reader and writer. Hence, readers of realist analytical texts can (and I do) read findings as partial, situated, and reflecting the positionality of the writer, of the reader (myself), and of the particular time and context in which the text was written and in which I read it. I do this even if (especially if) the author does not acknowledge her or his standpoint or impact on the findings. This problematizes Denzin's claim that traditional texts reproduce an image of the positivist reader and do not take into account the fact that readers "construct, apprehend, and bring meaning to and interact with the text in question" (p. 149). The text is not reproducing an image of its own; it needs the reader to be involved. I agree with Denzin that a text may offer more or fewer cues as to the type of reader it imagines (e.g., certainly medical journals offer more suggestions of a positivist reader than do medical humanities journals), but all texts are still open to different reading positions. I do not have to accept the position offered to me on the surface of an article; I can and do question assumptions of positivist or other analytic texts, just as I question the assumptions of stories and the power they reflect.

that is moved by and may move through, refract, and resist cultural inter-pretations. (p. 739)

Rather than simply the narrator or reporter of findings, I become in this account the main character of the story; this account is about my unique journey with the IOPOA.

As an autoethnographer, I have goals such as evocative writing of emo-tional experience (Ellis, 1997; Richardson, 2000), giving voice to topics tradi-tionally left out of social scientific inquiry (DeVault, 1990), producing writing of high literary/artistic quality (Ellis, 1997; Ellis & Bochner, 2000), and improving staff and patients' experience in health care (Ellingson, 1998). Autoethnography blurs the lines between sciences and humanities (e.g., Bochner, 1994; Bochner & Ellis, 1996; Ellis, 1997) and problematizes the dif-ferentiation between researcher and researched (DeVault, 1990; Ellis, Kiesinger, & Tillman-Healy, 1997; Fine, 1988; Mies, 1983; Reinharz, 1992).

Coffey (1999) proposed that ethnographers must reflect not only on how their presence in the field impacts on the lives of the people they are studying, but also on how the fieldwork experiences have affected the researcher's ongoing construction of self. The autoethnographic account in chapter 4 uses narrative and essay forms of writing blended together to reflect my personal sense-making process. As I wrote, I also was conscious of wanting to include my body in my story (see chap. 5 for a discussion of researcher embodiment).

Once I decided to write autoethnographically, I began thinking of events that were meaningful to me personally. I set my notes aside, and while I went back to them to find details, I did not hold myself to them as closely as I did with the narrative ethnography account. Jackson (1989) suggested that for researchers "our understanding of others can *only* proceed from within our own experience, and this experience involves our personalities and histories as much as our field research" (p. 17; italics original). I started with my emo-tional responses to the team members, patients, companions, and other can-cer center staff in constructing chapter 4 and used "writing as a method of inquiry" (Richardson, 2000). This account was enjoyable, but also deeply painful to write. I began chapter 4 with a vivid description of just how messed up my body was while I was completing early drafts of this project.

As I wrote my autoethnographic accounts, I noticed the presence of my body in the text—not just as a prop, but as central to how I came to under-stand the clinic—and this presence pointed to the absence of my body in the analytical portion of my book. I began to think about the huge piles of books, articles, reports, and essays in health communication theory and research that have taken over my desk throughout this project, almost none of which mentioned their authors' bodies.[3]

---

[3]In contrast, writing in disability studies often prominently features authors' bodies (e.g., Mairs, 1996; Zola, 1982).

Researchers have used the power of academic discourse to define their own bodies as essentially irrelevant to the production of knowledge. The performance of the "disembodied researcher" has been repeated for so long that it functions as a set of obscured, naturalized norms. We need to view researchers' bodies as sites for the production of knowledge about health communication. The invisibility of researchers' bodies in written accounts of health communication research limits our understandings of communication. Disembodied prose comes *from* nowhere, implying a disembodied author (Haraway, 1988).

The invisibility of researchers' bodies is a product of Cartesian dualism. Western cultures have continually reaffirmed the mind–body split and the association of the masculine with the mind and the feminine with the body (e.g., Spelman, 1999). Because the production of knowledge has traditionally been defined as the province of men, bodily knowledge has been systemically denied as oxymoronic. Indeed "it is as if 'facts' come out of our heads, and 'fictions' out of our bodies" (Simmonds, 1999, p. 52). Yet postcolonialist feminist theorist Trinh (1999) claimed that, "we do not *have* bodies, we *are* our bodies, and we are ourselves while being in the world. . . . We write— think and feel—(with) our bodies rather than only (with) our minds or hearts" (p. 258; italics original). Trinh's approach honors bodies as sources of knowledge and resists the mind–body division that is so pervasive in academia. For Trinh, the body is not a possession of higher mind to be manipulated and controlled to serve the purposes of the brain; the body and the person/self are one.

My (linguistically constructed and material) body is an essential aspect of my research process and of the academic tales I constructed. My perceptions of my body's gender, race, class, and sexual signifiers influenced my relationships in the field and my understanding of the standpoint from which I have written. The perceptions that team members, other clinic staff, patients, and patients' companions held about my body also affected our relationships. Ethnographer Coffey (1999) argued that fieldwork is an embodied practice, and the researcher's body—where it is positioned, what it looks like, what social groups or classifications it is perceived as belonging to—matters in the production of ethnographic accounts.

My body is most evident in the autoethnographic account, where I provide vivid descriptions of my body out of control. My experiences as a patient before and during my fieldwork rooted me physically in a patient perspective. I pointed out that writing while recovering from surgery made contemplation of my feelings and bodily experiences painful. Tales of my embodied experience in the clinic demystify the process of my research and writing. In the autoethnographic account, I demonstrate that my findings were as much the result of accidents, random occurrences, mistakes, and personal embarrassment as of carefully planned and executed methods (Foucault, 1977/1996). Including confessional or autobiographical accounts of the research process can function to strengthen the authenticity of accounts through their location of the researcher as an imperfect social actor (Coffey, 1999). The field of health communication is particularly appropriate as a site for research with embodied authors because of its focus on members of the "community of pain" (Frank, 1995), who are marked by bodily illness or injury. Patients and survivors frequently compose illness narratives to make sense of their experiences; using embodied narrative and autoethnographic methods and genres to explore patients' (narrative) constructions of meaning of their illness is clearly fitting (Frank, 1991, 1995).

Like the other two methodologies, autoethnography cannot accomplish all representational goals. In focusing on the researcher's experience, less attention is paid to others. Critics of autoethnography argue that it is self-indulgent, unscientific, and does not "count" as research (e.g., Atkinson, 1997). Because of the increased artistic license taken, narrative truth is privileged over empirically observed truth, and this is unacceptable to many social scientists. In addition, the wonderful details and specificity called for in the genre preclude some generalizations. Although readers ideally would identify with aspects of the story, the focus on an individual's experience seems to some to eliminate the possibility of generalizing to the experience of others. Other criticisms of autoethnography are similar to those of narrative—the narratives are still constructed by the author and hence do not diminish authorial power over representation. Autoethnographies make the researcher-author visible, but that visibility is carefully constructed, not neutral or innocent.

This genre offers embodied details, celebrates the author's position, problematizes the production of knowledge, and reveals the profane in the sacred processes of research. However, in not only exposing my positionality, but celebrating the uniqueness of my perspective, I make myself vulnerable to accusations of biased research that is invalid. Too much demystification can be politically dangerous. I acknowledge this risk, but I feel compelled to share my experience of research regardless. Those who would censure me for revealing the realities of research processes as I experienced them support a very different view of methodology than mine.

Appendix C

———◆———

CRYSTALLIZATION

As I moved back and forth between constructing narratives, writing personal reflections, and inductively deriving analytical categories and processes, I realized that I was playing with the constraints of the various genres and epistemologies by allowing each to inspire and shape the others; I was putting the modes of thinking and writing into conversation with one another. The narrative and autoethnographic accounts are informed by my inductive analysis of the data, in the sense that I developed a rough system of categories while I began drafting the narrative and autoethnographic accounts. The ideas of the processes that I wanted to include in the stories were in my mind as I constructed stories from notes and transcripts. I have been constructing narratives since my first month in the field. The narrative and autoethnographic accounts have as their goal to show the worlds of the clinic, which differs from my goal in the grounded theory analysis of "telling," of declaring my thoughts on how the team functions in the clinic. Thus, the storied accounts do not rest on claims of systematic analysis, but rather on claims of narrative truth and ethical responsibility to both honestly portray what I believe goes on there, and to do no harm to the people who shared their lives with me. At the same time, the narrative and autoethnographic accounts also affected the construction and representation of my grounded theory analysis. As I constructed stories, ideas and images came to me that resulted in further revision of my analytical schema, particularly in the noting of exceptions or less common events that I nonetheless considered vital to understanding the clinic.

The narrative at the beginning of this book, for example, shows the team acting together to deal with an emergency situation. A patient with severe cardiac distress is not a "typical event," but emergencies do arise periodically, and the ways in which the team members work together to address them reveal critical aspects of their individual personalities and ethic of care. After composing this narrative, I went back to my schema and rethought how emergency situations are part of the process of backstage communication I had described. Narratives also focused my attention on some events and diverted attention from others. Ordering events constructs meaning(s) for them, and these subsequent meanings affected my analytical process as well. I consider the reflexive relationship between my different forms of analysis and narrative representation to be a strength of my project. The use of different modes of writing calls attention to the constructed nature of all writing; readers experience the IOPOA team somewhat differently in each chapter. Both experimental and more traditional forms of social scientific writing reflect the power of the author to represent a world through words. The juxtaposition of complementary epistemologies becomes yet another facet of the crystal through which interpretation is encouraged.

LIMITATIONS OF CRYSTALLIZATION

Of course like any methodology or genre, there are some limitations to crystallization. First, not everyone is proficient in multiple genres and multiple forms of analysis. It is difficult and demanding to write evocative and engaging narrative alongside insightful, well-organized, and thoughtful analysis. Autoethnography can degenerate into exhibitionism or pointless self-indulgence. Analysis can be superficial. It takes a wide range of skills to do crystallization, and not many communication research programs exist that teach narrative writing as a method of analysis and representation.

Second, there is a trade-off between breadth and depth. In a single article or book, using crystallization enables an in-depth experience, but breath often is sacrificed for this depth. Strategic choices have to be made about what to center on because of space limitations. Embracing crystallization means other opportunities are forgone. Crystallization takes a lot of space and time.

Third, crystallization is not widely accepted as a viable methodology. Audiences often perceive of my project, for example, as self-contradictory and inconsistent. I encounter extreme opposition to my project despite repeated demonstration of the ability to write effectively in multiple genres. Many fields, such as medicine, do not welcome qualitative and interpretive methods, and crystallization is unlikely to be met with enthusiasm either. Indeed it may be even more threatening because it overtly denies the positivist paradigm while not embracing a single other standard of Truth either. The response to my work, although often positive, is just as often defensive, angry, and dismissive.

A fourth limitation is that researchers have to be willing to set aside or change their beliefs about the rightness or correctness of any given method or genre. They have to be willing to remember what is typically forgotten and often even consciously purged from published accounts—researchers make up generic and methodological standards, constraints, and practices. They are not sacred, pure science, nor sacred art; they are human constructions. Although I suspect most researchers know this on some level, it is quite a different matter to engage in genre and method play and have to overtly explore the degree to which all representations and practices are mere human constructions. This is not the same as having the skills to conduct good analyses and write in a given genre. Practitioners of crystallization have to have the courage to do so and the cognitive and emotional capacity to both suspend belief and implement it simultaneously. I have found such an exercise mentally invigorating, but it is also wearying and frustrating. Such a method leads to questions about epistemology, methodology, ethics, and even ontology of the researcher and her or his participants. At times the perpetual turning in on itself of the project feels like a descent into postmodern relativism. I do not think this is inevitable, and, ultimately, I believe my project avoids being mired such, but it is a demanding process for me personally and professionally.

References

Abramson, J. S., & Mizrahi, T. (1996). When social workers and physicians collaborate: Positive and negative interdisciplinary experiences. *Social Work, 41*, 270-281.

Ackerman, D. (1990). *A natural history of the senses.* New York: Random House.

Adelman, R. D., Greene, M. G., Charon, R., & Friedmann, E. (1990). Issues in the physician–geriatric patient relationship. In H. Giles, N. Coupland, & J. M. Wiemann (Eds.), *Communication, health, and the elderly* (pp. 126-134). London: Manchester University Press.

Adelman, R. D., Greene, M. G., Charon, R., & Friedmann, E. (1992). The content of physician and elderly patient interaction in the primary care encounter. *Communication Research, 19*, 370-380.

Allen, D. (1997). The nursing-medical boundary: A negotiated order? *Sociology of Health and Illness, 19*, 498-520.

Allen, D., Griffiths, L., Lyne, P., Monaghan, L., & De Murphy, D. (2002). Delivering health and social care: Changing roles, responsibilities and relationships. *Journal of Interprofessional Care, 16*, 79-80.

Applegate, W. B., Miller, S. T., Graney, M. J., Elam, J. T., Burns, R., & Akins, D. E. (1990). A randomized, controlled trial of a geriatric assessment unit in a community rehabilitation hospital. *New England Journal of Medicine, 322*, 1572-1578.

Arcangelo, V., Fitzgerald, M., Carroll, D., & Plumb, J. D. (1996). Collaborative care between nurse practitioners and primary care physicians. *Primary Care, 23*(1), 103-113.

Atkinson, P. (1995). *Medical talk and medical work.* Thousand Oaks, CA: Sage.

Atkinson, P. (1997). Narrative turn in a blind alley? *Qualitative Health Research, 7*, 325-344.

Barge, J. K., & Keyton, J. (1994). Contextualizing power and social influence in groups. In L. R. Frey (Ed.), *Group communication in context: Studies of natural groups* (pp. 85-106). Hillsdale, NJ: Lawrence Erlbaum Associates.

Barker, H. J., Williams, T. F., Zimmer, J. G., Van Buren, C., Vincent, S. J., & Pickrel, S. G. (1985). Geriatric consultation teams in acute hospitals: Impact on back-up of elderly patients. *Journal of American Geriatrics Society, 33*, 422-428.

Bateman, H., Bailey, P., & McLellan, H. (2003). Of rocks and safe channels: Learning to navigate as an interprofessional team. *Journal of Interprofessional Care, 17*, 141-150.

Battersby, C. (1999). Her body/her boundaries. In J. Price & M. Shildrick (Eds.), *Feminist theory and the body: A reader* (pp. 341-358). New York: Routledge.

Behar, R. (1995). Introduction: Out of exile. In R. Behar & D. A. Gordon (Eds.), *Women writing culture* (pp. 1-19). Berkeley: University of California Press.

Behar, R. (1996). *The vulnerable observer: Anthropology that breaks your heart*. Boston: Beacon.

Beisecker, A. E. (1990). Patient power in doctor–patient communication: What do we know? *Health Communication, 2,* 105-122.

Beisecker, A. E. (1996). Older persons' medical encounters and their outcomes. *Research On Aging, 18,* 9-31.

Berg, M. (1996). Practices of reading and writing: The constitutive role of the patient record in medical work. *Sociology of Health and Illness, 18,* 499-524.

Berger, P. L., & Luckmann, T. (1966). *The social construction of reality: A treatise in the sociology of knowledge*. New York: Doubleday.

Berteotti, C. R., & Seibold, D. R. (1994). Coordination and role-definition problems in health-care teams: A hospice case study. In L. R. Frey (Ed.), *Group communication in context: Studies of natural groups* (pp. 107-131). Hillsdale, NJ: Lawrence Erlbaum Associates.

Bochner, A. P. (1994). Perspectives on inquiry: II. Theories and stories. In M. Knapp & G. R. Miller (Eds.), *The handbook of interpersonal communication* (2nd ed., pp. 21-41). Thousand Oaks, CA: Sage.

Bochner, A. P. (1997). It's about time: Narrative and the divided self. *Qualitative Inquiry, 3,* 418-438.

Bochner, A. P., & Ellis, C. (1996). Introduction: Talking over ethnography. In C. Ellis & A. P. Bochner (Eds.), *Composing ethnography: Alternative forms of qualitative writing* (pp. 13-45). Walnut Creek, CA: AltaMira.

Bonsteel, A. (1997, March-April). Behind the white coat. *The Humanist, 57,* 15-19.

Borges, S., & Waitzkin, H. (1995). Women's narratives in primary medical care encounters. *Women and Health, 23,* 29-56.

Borisoff, D., & Merrill, L. (1992). *The power to communicate: Gender differences as barriers* (2nd. ed.). Prospect Heights, IL: Waveland.

Brody, H. (1992). *The healer's power*. New Haven, CT: Yale University Press.

Burl, J. B., Bonner, A., Rao, M., & Khan, A. M. (1998). Geriatric nurse practitioners in long-term care: Demonstration of effectiveness in managed care. *Journal of the American Geriatric Society, 46,* 506-510.

Butler, J. (1997). *Excitable speech: A politics of the performative*. New York: Routledge.

Campbell-Heider, N., & Pollack, D. (1987). Barriers to physician/nurse collegiality: An anthropological perspective. *Social Science and Medicine, 25,* 421-425.

Charmaz, K. (1990). "Discovering" chronic illness: Using grounded theory. *Social Science and Medicine, 30,* 1161-1172.

Charmaz, K. (2000). Grounded theory: Objectivist and constructivist methods. In N. K. Denzin & Y. S. Lincoln (Eds.), *Handbook of qualitative research* (2nd ed., pp. 509-535). Thousand Oaks, CA: Sage.

Clark, P. (1994). Social, professional and educational values on the interdisciplinary team: Implications for gerontological and geriatric education. *Educational Gerontology, 20,* 53-61.

Clough, P. T. (1994). *Feminist thought: Desire, power, and academic discourse*. Cambridge, MA: Blackwell.

Coffey, A. (1999). *The ethnographic self: Fieldwork and the representation of identity*. Thousand Oaks, CA: Sage.

Cooke, C. (1997). Reflections on the health care team: My experiences in an interdisciplinary program. *The Journal of the American Medical Association, 277,* 1091.

Cooley, E. (1994). Training an interdisciplinary team in communication and decision-making skills. *Small Group Research, 25,* 5-25.

Cott, C. (1998). Structure and meaning in multidisciplinary teamwork. *Sociology of Health and Illness, 20,* 848-873.

Cowen, D. L. (1992). Changing relationships between pharmacists and physicians. *American Journal of Hospital Pharmacy, 49,* 2715-2721.

Denzin, N. K. (1997). *Interpretive ethnography: Ethnographic practices for the 21st century.* Thousand Oaks, CA: Sage.

Denzin, N. K., & Lincoln, Y. S. (2000). Introduction: The discipline and practice of qualitative research. In N. K. Denzin & Y. S. Lincoln (Eds.), *Handbook of qualitative research* (2nd ed., pp. 1–28). Thousand Oaks, CA: Sage.

DeVault, M. L. (1990). Talking and listening from women's standpoint: Feminist strategies for interviewing and analysis. *Social Problems, 37,* 96-116.

Dollar, M. J., & Merrigan, G. M. (2002). Ethnographic practices in group communication research. In L. R. Frey (Ed.), *New directions in group communication* (pp. 59-78). Thousand Oaks, CA: Sage.

Donnelly, W. J. (1988). Righting the medical record: Transforming chronicle into story. *Journal of the American Medical Association, 260,* 823-825.

du Pre, A. (1999). *Communicating about health: Current issues and perspectives.* Mountain View, CA: Mayfield.

Edwards, J., & Smith, P. (1998). Impact of interdisciplinary education in underserved areas: Health professions collaboration in Tennessee. *Journal of Professional Nursing, 14,* 144-149.

Ehrenreich, B., & English, D. (1973). *Witches, midwives, and nurses: A history of women healers.* New York: Feminist Press.

Ellingson, L. L. (1998). "Then you know how I feel": Empathy, identification, and reflexivity in fieldwork. *Qualitative Inquiry, 4,* 492-514.

Ellingson, L. L. (2000, November). *The role of companions in the geriatric oncology patient-multidisciplinary health care provider interaction.* Paper presented at the National Communication Association, Seattle, WA.

Ellingson, L. L. (2002). The roles of companions in the geriatric oncology patient-interdisciplinary health care provider interaction. *Journal of Aging Studies, 16,* 361-382.

Ellingson, L. L., & Buzzanell, P. B. (1999). Listening to women's narratives of breast cancer treatment: A feminist approach to patient satisfaction with physician–patient communication. *Health Communication, 11,* 153-183.

Ellis, C. (1997). Evocative autoethnography: Writing emotionally about our lives. In W. Tierney & Y. Lincoln (Eds.), *Representation and the text: Reframing the narrative voice* (pp. 115-139). Albany: SUNY Press.

Ellis., C., & Bochner, A. P. (2000). Autoethnography, personal narrative, reflexivity: Researcher as subject. In N. K. Denzin & Y. S. Lincoln (Eds.), *Handbook of qualitative research* (2nd ed., pp. 733-768). Thousand Oaks, CA: Sage.

Ellis, C., Kiesinger, C. E., & Tillman-Healy, L. M. (1997). Interactive interviewing: Talking about emotional experience. In R. Hertz (Ed.), *Reflexivity and voice* (pp. 119-149). Thousand Oaks, CA: Sage.

Estes, Jr., E. H. (1981). The team context. In M. R. Haug (Ed.), *Elderly patients and their doctors* (pp. 132-136). New York: Springer.

Fagin, C. M. (1992). Collaboration between nurses and physicians: No longer a choice. *Academic Medicine, 67,* 295-303.

Ferguson, K. E. (1984). *The feminist case against bureaucracy.* Philadelphia: Temple University Press.

Ferguson, K. E. (1993). *The man question: Visions of subjectivity in feminist theory.* Berkeley: University of California Press.

Fine, M. G. (1988). What makes it feminist? *Women's Studies in Communication, 11,* 18-19.

Fischer, M. H., Martin Henry Fischer quotes. Retrieved on 12/30/03 from http://www.brainyquote.com/quotes/authors/m/martinhenr130015.html

Fisher, S. (1986). *In the patient's best interest: Women and the politics of medical decisions.* New Brunswick, NJ: Rutgers University Press.

Foucault, M. (1973/1994). *The birth of the clinic: An archaeology of medical perception* (A. M. S. Smith, Trans.). New York: Vintage Books.

Foucault, M. (1975/1995). *Discipline and punish: The birth of the prison* (A. Sheridan, Trans.). New York: Vintage Books.

Foucault, M. (1977/1996). Nietzsche, genealogy, history (D. Bouchard & S. Simon, Trans.). In L. E. Cahoone (Ed.), *From modernism to postmodernism: An anthology* (pp. 360-381). Cambridge, MA: Blackwell.

Fox, K. V. (1996). Silent voices: A subversive reading of child sexual abuse. In C. Ellis & A. P. Bochner (Eds.), *Composing ethnography: Alternative forms of qualitative writing* (pp. 330-356). Walnut Creek, CA: AltaMira.

Frank, A. W. (1991). Cancer self-healing: Health as cultural capital in monological society. *Studies in Symbolic Interaction, 12,* 105-222.

Frank, A. W. (1995). *The wounded storyteller: Body, illness, and ethics.* Chicago: University of Chicago Press.

Frey, L. R. (1994). *Group communication in context: Studies of natural groups.* Hillsdale, NJ: Lawrence Erlbaum Associates.

Furnham, A., Pendleton, D., & Manicom, C. (1981). The perception of different occupations within the medical profession. *Social Science and Medicine, 15,* 289-300.

Gabbard-Alley, A. S. (1995). Health communication and gender: A review and critique. *Health Communication, 7,* 35-54.

Gage, M. (1998). From independence to interdependence: Creating synergistic healthcare teams. *Journal of Nursing Administration, 28*(4), 17-26.

Garner, J. D. (1999). Feminism and feminist gerontology. In J. D. Garner (Ed.), *Fundamentals of feminist gerontology* (pp. 3-12). New York: Haworth.

Geertz, C. (1973). *The interpretation of cultures: Selected essays.* New York: Basic Books.

Geist-Martin, P., Ray, E. B., & Sharf, B. F. (2003). *Communicating health: Personal, cultural, and political complexities.* Belmont, CA: Wadsworth.

Gergen, K. J. (1994). *Realities and relationships: Soundings in social construction.* Cambridge, MA: Harvard University Press.

Glaser, B. G., (1992). *Basics of grounded theory analysis: Emergence vs. forcing.* Mill Valley, CA: Sociology Press.

Glaser, B., & Strauss, B. (1967). *The discovery of grounded theory: Strategies for qualitative research.* Chicago: Aldine.

Goffman, E. (1959). *The presentation of self in everyday life.* Garden City, NY: Doubleday.

Goodwin, M.H. (2002). Building power asymmetries in girls' interaction. *Discourse & Society, 13*, 715-730.

Griffiths, L. (1998). Humour as resistance to professional dominance in community mental health teams. *Sociology of Health and Illness, 20*, 874-895.

Gürsoy, A. (1996). Beyond the orthodox: Heresy in medicine and the social sciences from a cross-cultural perspective. *Social Science and Medicine, 43*, 577-599.

Hammick, M., Barr, H., Freeth, D., Koppel, I., & Reeves, S. (2002). Systematic review of evaluations of interprofessional education: Results and work in progress. *Journal of Interprofessional Care, 16*, 80-84.

Hannay, D. R. (1980). Problems of role identification and conflict in multidisciplinary teams. In J. H. Barber & C. R. Kratz (Eds.), *Towards team care* (pp. 3-17). Edinburgh: Churchill Livingstone.

Haraway, D. (1988). Situated knowledges: The science question in feminism and the privilege of partial perspective. *Feminist Studies, 14*, 575-599.

Haug, M. R. (1988). Professional client relationships and the older patient. In S. K. Steinmetz (Ed.), *Family and support systems across the life span* (pp. 225-242). New York: Plenum.

Haug, M. R. (1996). Elements in physician/patient interactions in late life. *Research on Aging, 18*, 32-51.

Hind, M., Norman, I., Cooper, S., Gill, E., Hilton, R., Judd, P., & Jones, S. C. (2003). Interprofessional perceptions of health care students. *Journal of Interprofessional Care, 17*, 21-34.

Hinojosa, J., Bedell, G., Buchholz, E. S., Charles, J., Shigaki, I. S., & Bicchieri, S.M. (2001). *Qualitative Health Research, 11*, 206-220.

Hummert, M. L., & Nussbaum, J. F. (Eds.). (2001). *Aging, communication, and health: Linking research and practice for successful aging.* Mahwah, NJ: Lawrence Erlbaum Associates.

Iles, P. A., & Auluck, R. (1990). From organizational to interorganizational development in nursing practice: Improving the effectiveness of interdisciplinary teamwork and interagency collaboration. *Journal of Advanced Nursing, 15*, 50-58.

Interdisciplinary Health Education Panel of the National League for Nursing. (1998). Building community: Developing skills for interprofessional health professions education and relationship-centered care. *Nursing and Health Care Perspectives, 19*, 87-90.

Jackson, M. (1989). *Paths toward a clearing: Radical empiricism and the ethnographic inquiry.* Bloomington: Indiana University Press.

Jones, R. A. P. (1997). Multidisciplinary collaboration: Conceptual development as a foundation for patient-focused care. *Holistic Nursing Practice, 11*(3), 8-16.

Jones, S. H. (1998). Turning the kaleidoscope, re-visioning feminist ethnography. *Qualitative Inquiry, 4*, 421-441.

Katriel, T. (1990). "Griping" as a verbal ritual in some Israeli discourse. In D. Carbaugh (Ed.), *Cultural communication and intercultural contact* (pp. 99-117). Hillsdale, NJ: Lawrence Erlbaum Associates.

Katzman, E. M. (1989). Nurses' and physicians' perceptions of nursing authority. *Journal of Professional Nursing, 5*, 208-214.

King, S. (2000, June 19-26). On Impac. *The New Yorker, 76*(16), 78-86.

Kreps, G. L. (1980). A field experimental test and revaluation of Weick's model of organizing. In D. Nimmo (Ed.), *Communication yearbook 4* (pp. 384-398). New Brunswick, NJ: Transaction Press.

Kreps, G. L. (1988). The pervasive role of information in health and health care: Implications for health communication policy. In J. Anderson (Ed.), *Communication yearbook 11* (pp. 238-276). Newbury Park, CA: Sage.

Kreps, G. L. (1990). *Organizational communication: Theory and practice* (2nd ed.). New York: Longman.

Kreps, G. L., & Thornton, B. C. (1992). *Health communication: Theory and practice0...* (2nd ed.). Prospect Heights, IL: Waveland.

Kulys, R., & Davis, M., Sr. (1987). Nurses and social worker: Rivals in the provision of social services? *Health and Social Work, 12,* 101-112.

Laine-Timmerman, L. E. (1999). *Living the mystery: The emotional experience of floor nursing.* Unpublished doctoral dissertation, University of South Florida, Tampa, FL.

Lammers, J. C., & Krikorian, D. H. (1997). Theoretical extension and operationalization of the bona fide group construct with an application to surgical teams. *Journal of Applied Communication Research, 25,* 17-38.

Langhorne, P., Williams, B., Gilchrist, W., & Howie, K. (1993). Do stroke units save lives? *Lancet, 342,* 395-398.

Lengel, L. B. (1998). Researching the "other," transforming ourselves: Methodological considerations of feminist ethnography. *Journal of Communication Inquiry, 22,* 229-250.

Lesch, C. (1994). Observing theory in a practice: Sustaining consciousness in a coven. In L. R. Frey, (Ed.), *Group communication in context: Studies of natural groups* (pp. 57-82). Hillsdale, NJ: Lawrence Erlbaum.

Lichtenstein, R., Alexander, J. A., Jinnett, K., & Ullman, E. (1997). Embedded intergroup relations in interdisciplinary teams: Effects on perceptions of level of team integration. *Journal of Applied Behavioral Science, 33,* 413-434.

Lindlof, T. R., & Taylor, B. C. (2002). *Qualitative communication research methods* (2nd ed.). Thousand Oaks, CA: Sage.

Lingard, L., Reznick, R., DeVito, I., & Espin, S. (2002). Forming professional identities on the health care team: Discursive constructions of the "other" in the operating room. *Medical Education, 36,* 728-734.

Mairs, N. (1996). *Waist high in the world: A life among the nondisabled.* Boston: Beacon.

Mairs, N. (1997). Carnal acts. In K. Conboy, N. Medina, & S. Stanbury (Eds.), *Writing on the body: Female embodiment and feminist theory* (pp. 296-305). New York: Columbia University Press.

Mann, D. (1998, January 8). Doctors, patients need to talk more. *Medical Tribune (Family Physician Edition), 39*(1), 1, 6.

McCandless, N. J., & Conner, F. P. (1999). Older women and the health care system: A time for change. In J. D. Garner (Ed.), *Fundamentals of feminist gerontology* (pp. 13-27). New York: Haworth.

McClelland, M., & Sands, R. (1993). The missing voice in interdisciplinary communication. *Qualitative Health Research, 3,* 74-90.

McCormick, W. C., Inui, T. S., & Roter, D. L. (1996). Interventions in physician-elderly patient interactions. *Research on Aging, 18,* 103-136.

McHugh, M., West, P., Assatly, C., Duprat, L., Niloff, J., Waldo, K., Wandel, J., & Clifford, J. (1996). Establishing an interdisciplinary patient care team: Collaboration at the bedside and beyond. *Journal of Nursing Administration, 26*(4), 21-27.

Mellor, M. J., Hyer, K., & Howe, J. L. (2002). The geriatric interdisciplinary team approach: Challenges and opportunities in educating trainees together from a variety of disciplines. *Educational Gerontology, 28,* 867-880.

Meyers, R. A., & Brashers, D. E. (1994). Expanding the boundaries of small group communication research: Exploring a feminist perspective. *Communication Studies, 45,* 68-85.

Mies, M. (1983). Towards a methodology for feminist research. In G. Bowles & R. D. Klein (Eds.), *Theories of women's studies* (pp. 117-139). London: Routledge & Kegan Paul.

Miller, D. K., Morley, J. E., Rubenstein, L. Z., Pietruszka, F. M., & Strome, L. S. (1990). Formal geriatric assessment instruments and the care of older general medical outpatients. *Journal of the American Geriatrics Society, 38,* 645-651.

Miller, W. L., & Crabtree, B. F. (2000). Clinical research. In N. K. Denzin & Y. S. Lincoln (Eds.), *Handbook of qualitative research* (2nd ed., pp. 607-631). Thousand Oaks, CA: Sage.

Mishler, E. G. (1984). *The discourse of medicine: Dialectics of medical interviews.* Norwood, NJ: Ablex.

Mizrahi, T., & Abramson, J. (1994). Collaboration between social workers and physicians: An emerging typology. In E. Sherman & W. J. Reid (Eds.), *Qualitative research in social work* (pp. 135-151). New York: Columbia University Press.

Northrup, C. (1994). *Women's bodies, women's wisdom: Creating physical and emotional health and healing.* New York: Bantam.

Nursing 91. (1991, June). The nurse-doctor game. *Nursing 91, 21,* 60-64.

Olesen, V. L. (2000). Feminisms and qualitative research at and into the millennium. In N. K. Denzin & Y. S. Lincoln (Eds.), *Handbook of qualitative research* (2nd ed., pp. 215-255). Thousand Oaks, CA: Sage.

Opie, A. (1997). Thinking teams thinking clients: Issues of discourse and representation in the work of health care teams. *Sociology of Health and Illness, 19,* 259-280.

Opie, A. (1998). "Nobody's asked me for my view": Users' empowerment by multidisciplinary health teams. *Qualitative Health Research, 8,* 188-206.

Opie, A. (2000). *Thinking teams/thinking clients: Knowledge-based teamwork.* New York: Columbia University Press.

Pike, A. W. (1991). Moral outrage and moral discourse in nurse-physician collaboration. *Journal of Professional Nursing, 7,* 351-363.

Pincus, C. R. (1995). Why medicine is driving doctors crazy. *Medical Economics, 72,* 40-44.

Poole, M. S. (1990). Do we have any theories of communication? *Communication Studies, 41,* 237-247.

Poole, M. S. (1994). Breaking the isolation of small group communication research. *Communication Studies, 45,* 20-28.

Prescott, P. A., & Bowen, S. A. (1985). Physician–nurse relationships. *Annals of Internal Medicine, 103,* 127-133.

Propp, K. M., & Kreps, G. L. (1994). A rose by any other name: The vitality of group communication. *Communication Studies, 45,* 7-19.

Putnam, L. L. (1994). Revitalizing small group communication: Lessons learned from a small group perspective. *Communication Studies, 45,* 97-102.

Putnam, L. L., & Stohl, C. (1990). Bona fide groups: A reconceptualization of groups in context. *Communication Studies, 41,* 248-265.

Ray, R. E. (1996). A postmodern perspective on feminist gerontology. *The Gerontologist, 36*, 674-680.

Ray, R. E. (1999). Researching to transgress: The need for critical feminism in gerontology. In J. D. Garner (Ed.), *Fundamentals of feminist gerontology* (pp. 171-184). New York: Haworth.

Reinharz, S. (1992). *Feminist methods in social research.* New York: Oxford University Press.

Resnick, C. (1997). The role of multidisciplinary community clinics in managed care systems. *Social Work, 42*, 91-98.

Richardson, L. (1990). Narrative and sociology. *Journal of Contemporary Ethnography, 19*, 116-135.

Richardson, L. (1997). *Fields of play: Constructing an academic life.* New Brunswick, NJ: Rutgers University Press.

Richardson, L. (2000). Writing: A method of inquiry. In N. K. Denzin & Y. S. Lincoln (Eds.), *Handbook of qualitative research* (2nd ed., pp. 923-943). Thousand Oaks, CA: Sage.

Roter, D. L., Stewart, M., Putnam, S. M., Lipkin, Jr., M., Stiles, W., & Inui, T. S. (1997). Communication patterns of primary care physicians. *Journal of the American Medical Association, 277*, 350-357.

Rubenstein, L. Z., Abrass, I. B., & Kane, R. L. (1981). Improved care for geriatric patients on a new geriatric evaluation unit. *Journal of the American Geriatrics Society, 29*, 531-536.

Rubenstein, L. Z., Josephson, K. R., Wieland, G. D., English, P. A., Sere, J. A., & Kane, R. L. (1984). Effectiveness of a geriatric evaluation unit: A randomized clinical trial. *New England Journal of Medicine, 311*, 1664-1670.

Rubenstein, L. Z., Stuck, A. E., Siu, A. L., & Wieland, D. (1991). Impacts of geriatric evaluation and management programs on defined outcomes: Overview of the evidence. *Journal of the American Geriatrics Society, 39(Suppl.)*, 9S-16S.

Rubenstein, L. Z., Wieland, G. D., English, P. A., Josephson, K. R., Sere, J. A., & Abrass, I. B. (1984). The Sepulveda VA geriatric evaluation unit: Data on four-year outcomes and predictors of improved patient outcomes. *Journal of the American Geriatrics Society, 32*, 503-512.

Ryan, J. W. (1999, March-April). Collaboration of the nurse practitioner and physician in long-term care. *Lippincotts Primary Care Practitioner, 3*(2), 127-134.

Sacks, K. B. (1988). *Caring by the hour: Women, work, and organizing at Duke Medical Center.* Urbana: University of Illinois Press.

Sacks, O. (1984). *A leg to stand on.* New York: Simon & Schuster.

Saltz, C. (1992). The interdisciplinary team in geriatric rehabilitation. *Geriatric Social Work Education, 18*, 133-143.

Sands, R. (1993). "Can you overlap here?": A question for an interdisciplinary team. *Discourse Processes, 16*, 545-564.

Sands, R., Stafford, J., & McClelland, M. (1990). "I beg to differ": Conflict in the interdisciplinary team. *Social Work in Health Care, 14*(3), 55-72.

Satin, D. G. (1994). The interdisciplinary, integrated approach to professional practice with the aged. In D. G. Satin (Ed.), *The clinical care of the aged person: An interdisciplinary perspective* (pp. 391-403). New York: Oxford University Press.

Schmidt, I., Claesson, C. B., Westerholm, B., Nilsson, L. G., & Svarstad, B. L. (1998). The impact of multidisciplinary team interventions on psychotropic prescribing in Swedish nursing homes. *Journal of the American Geriatrics Society, 46*, 77-82.

Schmitt, M. H., Farrell, M. P., & Heinemann, G. D. (1988). Conceptual and methodological problems in studying the effects of interdisciplinary geriatric teams. *The
Gerontologist, 28,* 753-764.

Sheppard, M. (1992). Contact and collaboration with general practitioners: A comparison of social workers and psychiatric nurses. *British Journal of Social Work, 22,*
419-436.

Siegel, B. S. (1994). Developing interdisciplinary teams. In D. G. Satin (Ed.), *The clinical care of the aged person: An interdisciplinary perspective* (pp. 404-425). New
York: Oxford University Press.

Simmonds, F. N. (1999). My body, myself: How does a black woman do sociology? In
J. Price & M. Shildrick (Eds.), *Feminist theory and the body: A reader* (pp. 50-63).
New York: Routledge.

Spelman, E. V. (1999). Woman as body: Ancient and contemporary views. In J. Price
& M. Shildrick (Eds.), *Feminist theory and the body: A reader* (pp. 31-41). New
York: Routledge.

Stack, C. B. (1993). Writing ethnography: Feminist critical practice. *Frontiers, 13*(3),
77-89.

Starhawk. (1988). *Dreaming the dark: Magic, sex and politics, new edition.* Boston:
Beacon.

Stein, L. I. (1967). The doctor-nurse game. *Archives of General Psychiatry, 16,* 699-703.

Stein, L. I. (1990). The doctor-nurse game revisited. *The New England Journal of
Medicine, 322,* 546-549.

Stewart, J., & Logan, C. (1998), *Together: Communication interpersonally* (5th ed.).
Boston: McGraw-Hill.

Strauss, A. L., & Corbin, J. (1990). *Basics of qualitative research: Grounded theory procedures and techniques.* Newbury Park, CA: Sage.

Strauss, A. L., & Corbin, J. (1998). *Basics of qualitative research: Grounded theory procedures and techniques* (2nd ed.). Newbury Park, CA: Sage.

Sullivan, P. A., & Fisher, P. S. (1995). Challenges in a multidisciplinary head and neck
oncology program. *Cancer Practice, 3,* 258-260.

Tannen, D. (1990). *You just don't understand: Women and men in conversation.* New
York: Ballantine.

Tedlock, B. (1991). From participant observation to the observation of participation:
The emergence of narrative ethnography. *Journal of Anthropological Research, 41,*
69-94.

Trella, R. S. (1993). A multidisciplinary approach to case management of frail, hospitalized older adults. *Journal of Nursing Administration, 23*(2), 20-26.

Trinh, T. M. (1999). Write your body: The body in theory. In J. Price & M. Shildrick
(Eds.), *Feminist theory and the body: A reader* (pp. 258-266). New York: Routledge.

Turner, P., Sheldon, F., Coles, C., Mountford, B., Hillier, R., Radway, P., & Wee, B.
(2000). Listening to and learning from the family carer's story: An innovative
approach in interprofessional education. *Journal of Interprofessional Care, 14,*
387-395.

Vanderford, M. L., Jenks, E. B., & Sharf, B. F. (1997). Exploring patients' experiences
as a primary source of meaning. *Health Communication, 9,* 13-26.

Van Maanen, J. (1988). *Tales of the field: On writing ethnography.* Chicago: University
of Chicago Press.

Vroman, K., & Kovacich, J. (2002). Computer-mediated interdisciplinary teams:
Theory and reality. *Journal of Interprofessional Care, 16,* 159-170.

Waitzkin, H. (1984). Doctor–patient communication. *Journal of the American Medical Association, 252,* 2441-2446.

Wear, D. (1997). *Privilege in the medical academy: A feminist examines gender, race, and power.* New York: Teachers College Press.

Weick, K. E. (1969). *The social psychology of organizing.* Reading, MA: Addison-Wesley.

Wieland, D., Kramer, B. J., Waite, M. S., & Rubenstein, L. Z. (1996). The interdisciplinary team in geriatric care. *American Behavioral Scientist, 39,* 655-664.

Williams, A. (1993). Diversity and agreement in feminist ethnography. *Sociology, 27,* 575-589.

Williams, M. E., Williams, T. F., Zimmer, J. G., Hall, W. J., & Podgorski, M. S. (1987). How does the team approach to outpatient geriatric evaluation compare with traditional care: A report of a randomized controlled trial. *Journal of the American Geriatric Society, 35,* 1071-1078.

Williams, S. J., & Calnan, M. (1996). The "limits" of medicalization?: Modern medicine and the lay populace in "late" modernity. *Social Science and Medicine, 42,* 1609-1620.

Wolf, M. (1992). *A thrice told tale: Feminism, postmodernism, and ethnographic responsibility.* Stanford, CA: Stanford University Press.

Wood, J. T. (1994). Engendered identities: Shaping voice and mind through gender. In D. R. Vocate (Ed.), *Intrapersonal communication: Different voices, different minds* (pp. 145-167). Hillsdale, NJ: Lawrence Erlbaum Associates.

Wood, J. T. (2005). *Gendered lives: Communication, gender, and culture* (6th ed.). Belmont, CA: Wadsworth.

Wood, J. T., McMahan, E. M., & Stacks, D. W. (1984). Research on women's communication: Critical assessment and recommendations. In D. L. Fowlkes & C. S. McClure (Eds.), *Feminist visions: Toward a transformation of the liberal arts curriculum* (pp. 31-41). Tuscaloosa: University of Alabama Press.

Wyatt, N. (1991). Physician–patient relationships: What do doctors say? *Health Communication, 3,* 157-174.

Wyatt, N. (1993). Organizing and relating: Feminist critique of small group communication. In S. P. Bowen & N. Wyatt (Eds.), *Transforming visions: Feminist critiques in communication studies* (pp. 51-86). Cresskill, NJ: Hampton.

Wyatt, N. (2002). Foregrounding feminist theory in group communication research. In L. R. Frey (Ed.), *New directions in group communication* (pp. 43-56). Thousand Oaks, CA: Sage.

Zimmer, J. G., Groth-Junker, A., & McClusker, J. (1985). A randomized controlled study of a home health care team. *American Journal of Public Health, 75,* 134-141.

Zola, I. K. (1982). *Missing pieces: A chronicle of living with a disability.* Philadelphia: Temple University Press.

Zola, I. K. (1990). Medicine as an institution of social control. In P. Conrad & R. Kern (Eds.), *The sociology of health and illness: Critical perspectives* (3rd ed., pp. 398-408). New York: St. Martin's Press.

About the Author

Laura L. Ellingson (Ph.D., University of South Florida) is an Assistant Professor in the Department of Communication at Santa Clara University. Her research interests include health care provider–patient communication, interdisciplinary communication, health care teamwork, communication and gender, and feminist theory and methodology. Her publications include articles in *Health Communication*, *Journal of Aging Studies*, *Journal of Applied Communication Research*, *Women's Studies in Communication*, and *Communication Studies*. She has served as Chair of the Ethnography Division of the National Communication Association. Currently, she is conducting an ethnography of team communication in a dialysis clinic.

Author Index

Subject Index

CPSIA information can be obtained
at www.ICGtesting.com
Printed in the USA
BVHW07s2309240718
522554BV00002B/174/P